Ear Implants

Editors

COLIN L. DRISCOLL
BRIAN A. NEFF

OTOLARYNGOLOGIC CLINICS OF NORTH AMERICA

www.oto.theclinics.com

December 2014 • Volume 47 • Number 6

ELSEVIER

1600 John F. Kennedy Boulevard • Suite 1800 • Philadelphia, Pennsylvania, 19103-2899

http://www.oto.theclinics.com

OTOLARYNGOLOGIC CLINICS OF NORTH AMERICA Volume 47, Number 6
December 2014 ISSN 0030-6665, ISBN-13: 978-0-323-34042-7

Editor: Joanne Husovski
Developmental Editor: Susan Showalter

Otolaryngologic Clinics of North America (ISSN 0030-6665) is published bimonthly by Elsevier, Inc., 360 Park Avenue South, New York, NY 10010-1710. Months of issue are February, April, June, August, October, and December. Business and Editorial Offices: 1600 John F. Kennedy Blvd., Suite 1800, Philadelphia, PA 19103-2899. Customer Service Office: 6277 Sea Harbor Drive, Orlando, FL 32887-4800. Periodicals postage paid at New York, NY and additional mailing offices. Subscription prices is $365.00 per year (US individuals), $692.00 per year (US institutions), $175.00 per year (US student/resident), $485.00 per year (Canadian individuals), $876.00 per year (Canadian institutions), $540.00 per year (international individuals), $876.00 per year (international institutions), $270.00 per year (international & Canadian student/resident). Foreign air speed delivery is included in all *Clinics'* subscription prices. All prices are subject to change without notice. **POSTMASTER:** Send address changes to *Otolaryngologic Clinics of North America*, Elsevier Health Sciences Division, Subscription Customer Service, 3251 Riverport Lane, Maryland Heights, MO 63043. **Telephone: 1-800-654-2452 (U.S. and Canada); 314-447-8871 (outside U.S. and Canada). Fax: 314-447-8029. E-mail: journalscustomerservice-usa@elsevier.com (for print support); journalsonlinesupport-usa@elsevier.com (for online support).**

Reprints. For copies of 100 or more of articles in this publication, please contact the Commercial Reprints Department, Elsevier Inc., 360 Park Avenue South, New York, NY 10010-1710. Tel.: 212-633-3874; Fax: 212-633-3820; E-mail: reprints@elsevier.com.

Otolaryngologic Clinics of North America is also published in Spanish by McGraw-Hill Interamericana Editores S.A., P.O. Box 5-237, 06500 Mexico D.F., Mexico.

Otolaryngologic Clinics of North America is covered in *MEDLINE/PubMed (Index Medicus), Current Contents/Clinical Medicine, Excerpta Medica, BIOSIS, Science Citation Index,* and *ISI/BIOMED.*

PROGRAM OBJECTIVE
The goal of the *Otolaryngologic Clinics of North America* is to provide information on the latest trends in patient management, the newest advances; and provide a sound basis for choosing treatment options in the field of otolaryngology.

TARGET AUDIENCE
All practicing physicians and healthcare professionals who provide patient care to otolaryngologic patients.

LEARNING OBJECTIVES
Upon completion of this activity, participants will be able to:
1. Describe sound mechanics of implantable hearing devices.
2. Discuss the development of active middle ear hearing implant.
3. Vibrant soundbridge rehabilitation of mixed and conductive as well as sensorineural hearing loss.

ACCREDITATION
The Elsevier Office of Continuing Medical Education (EOCME) is accredited by the Accreditation Council for Continuing Medical Education (ACCME) to provide continuing medical education for physicians.

The EOCME designates this enduring material for a maximum of 15 *AMA PRA Category 1 Credit*(s)™. Physicians should claim only the credit commensurate with the extent of their participation in the activity.

All other health care professionals requesting continuing education credit for this enduring material will be issued a certificate of participation.

DISCLOSURE OF CONFLICTS OF INTEREST
The EOCME assesses conflict of interest with its instructors, faculty, planners, and other individuals who are in a position to control the content of CME activities. All relevant conflicts of interest that are identified are thoroughly vetted by EOCME for fair balance, scientific objectivity, and patient care recommendations. EOCME is committed to providing its learners with CME activities that promote improvements or quality in healthcare and not a specific proprietary business or a commercial interest.

The planning committee, staff, authors and editors listed below have identified no financial relationships or relationships to products or devices they or their spouse/life partner have with commercial interest related to the content of this CME activity:
Thomas Beleites, MD; Matthias Bornitz, PhD; Matthew L. Carlson, MD; Kristen Helm; Brynne Hunter; Joanne Husovski; Karl-Bernd Hüttenbrink, MD; Herman A. Jenkins, MD; Andleeb Khan, MD; Sandy Lavery; Jan-Christoffer Lüers, MD; Sam J. Marzo, MD; Jill McNair; Brian A. Neff, MD; Marcus Neudert, MD; Stanley Pelosi, MD; Santha Priya; Joshua M. Sappington, MD; Susan Showalter; Kristin Uhler, PhD; Thomas Zahnert, MD.

The planning committee, staff, authors and editors listed below have identified financial relationships or relationships to products or devices they or their spouse/life partner have with commercial interest related to the content of this CME activity:
Douglas Chen, MD, FACS is a consultant/advisor for Med-El.
Colin L. Driscoll, MD is a consultant/advisor for Cochlear Ltd.
Michael E. Glasscock, III, MD is on speakers bureau, is a consultant/advisor, has stock ownership and research grants from Ototronix LLC, Otomed, Inc., and Envoy Medical; also has employment affiliation and royalties/patents with Otomed, Inc.
David S. Haynes, MD, FACS is a consultant/advisor for Cochlear Ltd., Med-El, Advanced Bionics AG, Stryker, ANSPACH/Synthes and Grace Medical
Todd Hillman, MD is a consultant/advisor for Med-El.
Jack A. Shohet, MD is a consultant/advisor for Envoy Medical.

UNAPPROVED/OFF-LABEL USE DISCLOSURE
The EOCME requires CME faculty to disclose to the participants:
1. When products or procedures being discussed are off-label, unlabelled, experimental, and/or investigational (not US Food and Drug Administration [FDA] approved); and
2. Any limitations on the information presented, such as data that are preliminary or that represent ongoing research, interim analyses, and/or unsupported opinions. Faculty may discuss information about pharmaceutical agents that is outside of FDA-approved labelling. This information is intended solely for CME and is not intended to promote off-label use of these medications. If you have any questions, contact the medical affairs department of the manufacturer for the most recent prescribing information.

TO ENROLL
To enroll in the *Otolaryngologic Clinics of North America* Continuing Medical Education program, call customer service at 1-800-654-2452 or sign up online at http://www.theclinics.com/home/cme. The CME program is available to subscribers for an additional annual fee of USD 260.

METHOD OF PARTICIPATION
In order to claim credit, participants must complete the following:
1. Complete enrolment as indicated above.
2. Read the activity.
3. Complete the CME Test and Evaluation. Participants must achieve a score of 70% on the test. All CME Tests and Evaluations must be completed online.

CME INQUIRIES/SPECIAL NEEDS
For all CME inquiries or special needs, please contact elsevierCME@elsevier.com.

Contributors

EDITORS

COLIN L. DRISCOLL, MD
Professor and Chair, Department of Otorhinolaryngology, Mayo Clinic, Rochester, Minnesota

BRIAN A. NEFF, MD
Assistant Professor and Consultant, Department of Otorhinolaryngology, Mayo Clinic, Rochester, Minnesota

AUTHORS

THOMAS BELEITES, MD
Department of Medicine, Clinic of Otorhinolaryngology, Technische Universität Dresden, Dresden, Germany

MATTHIAS BORNITZ, PhD
Department of Medicine, Clinic of Otorhinolaryngology, Technische Universität Dresden, Dresden, Germany

MATTHEW L. CARLSON, MD
Assistant Professor, Department of Otolaryngology-Head and Neck Surgery, Mayo Clinic, Rochester, Minnesota; Clinical Fellow, Department of Otolaryngology, Vanderbilt University Medical Center, Nashville, Tennessee

DOUGLAS CHEN, MD
Pittsburgh Ear Associates, Pittsburgh, Pennsylvania

MICHAEL E. GLASSCOCK III, MD
Clinical Professor Emeritus, Department of Otolaryngology, Vanderbilt University Medical Center, Nashville, Tennessee

DAVID S. HAYNES, MD
Department of Otolaryngology-Head and Neck Surgery, The Bill Wilkerson Center for Otolaryngology and Communication Sciences, Vanderbilt University, Nashville, Tennessee

TODD HILLMAN, MD
Pittsburgh Ear Associates, Pittsburgh, Pennsylvania

KARL-BERND HÜTTENBRINK, MD
Professor, Department of Otorhinolaryngology, Head and Neck Surgery, University of Cologne, Cologne, Germany

HERMAN A. JENKINS, MD
Professor and Chair, Otolaryngology, University of Colorado, School of Medicine, Aurora, Colorado

ANDLEEB KHAN, MD
Pittsburgh Ear Associates, Pittsburgh, Pennsylvania

JAN-CHRISTOFFER LÜERS, MD
Associate Professor, Department of Otorhinolaryngology, Head and Neck Surgery,
University of Cologne, Cologne, Germany

SAM J. MARZO, MD
Department of Otolaryngology-Head and Neck Surgery, Loyola University Medical
Center, Maywood, Illinois

MARCUS NEUDERT, MD
Department of Medicine, Clinic of Otorhinolaryngology, Technische Universität Dresden,
Dresden, Germany

STANLEY PELOSI, MD
Assistant Professor, Department of Otolaryngology, The New York Eye and Ear Infirmary,
New York, New York; Assistant Professor, Department of Otolaryngology-Head and Neck
Surgery, Thomas Jefferson University, Philadelphia, Pennsylvania

JOSHUA M. SAPPINGTON, MD
Department of Otolaryngology-Head and Neck Surgery, Loyola University Medical
Center, Maywood, Illinois

JACK A. SHOHET, MD
Shohet Ear Associates, New Port Beach, California

KRISTIN UHLER, PhD
Assistant Professor, Department of Otolaryngology, University of Colorado, School of
Medicine, Aurora, Colorado

THOMAS ZAHNERT, MD
Professor, Department of Medicine, Clinic of Otorhinolaryngology, Technische Universität
Dresden, Dresden, Germany

Contents

Implantable hearing aids are gaining importance for the treatment of sensorineural hearing loss and also for mixed hearing loss. The various hearing aid systems, combined with different middle ear situations, give rise to a wide range of different reconstructions. This article attempts to summarize the current knowledge concerning the mechanical interaction between active middle ear implants (AMEIs) and the normal or reconstructed middle ear. Some basic characteristics of the different AMEIs are provided in conjunction with the middle ear mechanics. The interaction of AMEIs and middle ear and the influence of various boundary conditions are discussed in more detail.

Active middle ear implants (AMEIs) are sophisticated technologies designed to overcome many of the shortcomings of conventional hearing aids, including feedback, distortion, and occlusion effect. Three AMEIs are currently approved by the US Food and Drug Administration for implantation in patients with sensorineural hearing loss. In this article, the history of AMEI technologies is reviewed, individual component development is outlined, past and current implant systems are described, and design and implementation successes and dead ends are highlighted. Past and ongoing challenges facing AMEI development are reviewed.

The Vibrant Soundbridge is the world's most often implanted active middle ear implant or hearing aid. During the last few years, the device indications have expanded from sensorineural hearing loss to conductive and mixed hearing loss. Titanium couplers have led to improved contact of the floating mass transducer with the middle ear structures. The resulting hearing gain is satisfying for most patients, but so far, there is no clear audiologic advantage over conventional hearing aids. Currently, the indications are mainly related to intolerance of conventional hearing aids (eg, chronic otitis externa), severe mixed hearing loss with a destructed middle ear and certain medical diagnosis (eg, congenital atresia).

The Vibrant Soundbridge is a means to rehabilitate patients with sensorineural hearing loss. It differs from hearing aids in that it uses mechanical

losses in animal and human cadaveric models. These devices are in their infancy, and further study is needed to better identify candidates and develop appropriate expectations.

OTOLARYNGOLOGIC CLINICS OF NORTH AMERICA

Preface

Ear Implants

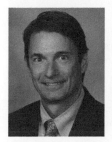 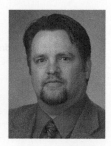

Colin L. Driscoll, MD   Brian A. Neff, MD
Editors

It has been our distinct pleasure to work with such a fine group of authors to explore the current state of active middle ear implants. We thank them for the comprehensive yet clinically relevant and succinct presentations. Partially and totally implantable hearing rehabilitation devices have gained widespread acceptance by physicians and patients, particularly cochlear implants and osseointegrated implants. This issue of *Otolaryngologic Clinics of North America* explores the evolving world of active middle ear implants.

The development of this technology has been slow and challenging, and in this issue, we explore the history of device development to aid in understanding what has led to successful platforms. Experts with extensive personal knowledge of the technology and outcomes review all of the current FDA-approved devices in detail. We asked for and received an objective assessment of each device. There are little peer-reviewed data on which to rely, and thus, a necessary role for expert opinion.

The knowledge of physicians and expertise of engineers working creatively together are critical to the advancement of this exciting field, melding human and device. The discipline has advanced far enough that these devices and their future iterations will be a part of our armamentarium to combat hearing loss.

Colin L. Driscoll, MD
Department of Otorhinolaryngology
Mayo Clinic
Rochester, MN, USA

Brian A. Neff, MD
Department of Otorhinolaryngology
Mayo Clinic
Rochester, MN, USA

E-mail addresses:
driscoll.colin@mayo.edu (C.L. Driscoll)
Neff.Brian@mayo.edu (B.A. Neff)

Otolaryngol Clin N Am 47 (2014) xi
http://dx.doi.org/10.1016/j.otc.2014.09.016
0030-6665/14/$ – see front matter © 2014 Elsevier Inc. All rights reserved.

Sound Transfer of Active Middle Ear Implants

Thomas Beleites, MD, Marcus Neudert, MD, Matthias Bornitz, PhD,
Thomas Zahnert, MD*

KEYWORDS

- Active middle ear implant • Transfer function • Vibroplasty • Middle ear
- Reconstruction • Ossicular chain

KEY POINTS

- Larger contact area between transducer and ossicular chain improves coupling.
- Ensure a tight and stable contact between the actuator and the ossicle (cartilage, coupling devices with bell or clip mechanisms).
- Floating mass transducer movement axis has to be in an orthogonal (perpendicular) projection to the round window membrane plane.
- Vibroplasty with direct coupling to the inner ear fluid should only be used in cases of noncontaminated middle ear.

INTRODUCTION

Implantable hearing aids are gaining importance not only for the treatment of sensorineural hearing loss but also for mixed hearing loss. The various hearing aid systems, combined with different middle ear situations, give rise to a wide range of different reconstructions. The actuators of the implantable hearing aids, also referred to as active middle ear implants (AMEIs), and the middle ear form one mechanically interacting system (the term AMEI is used synonymously for the actuator and the complete implantable hearing aid). Understanding the mechanical characteristics of this system and the interactions is a prerequisite for explaining and improving the results of active middle ear reconstructions.

The tympanic membrane and the connected ossicular chain with joints and ligaments are the natural part of this mechanical system. In recent years, knowledge about the normal function of the middle ear has improved thanks to optical laser Doppler vibrometry (LDV) measurements on animal and temporal bone models. The frequency-dependent 3-dimensional vibration patterns of the tympanic membrane and ossicular chain have been demonstrated in many publications and are widely

Department of Medicine, Clinic of Otorhinolaryngology, Technische Universität Dresden, Fetscherstrasse 74, Dresden 01307, Germany
* Corresponding author.
E-mail address: Thomas.zahnert@uniklinikum-dresden.de

Otolaryngol Clin N Am 47 (2014) 859–891
http://dx.doi.org/10.1016/j.otc.2014.08.001
oto.theclinics.com

Abbreviations	
AMEI	Active middle ear implant
DACS	Direct acoustic cochlear stimulator
eq.	Equivalent
FEM	Finite element model
FMT	Floating mass transducer
GME	Middle-ear pressure gain
LDV	Laser Doppler vibrometry
METF	Middle ear transfer function
PORP	Partial ossicular replacement prosthesis
RW	Round window
RWM	Round window membrane
SPL	Sound pressure level
STF	Sound transfer function
TF	Transfer function
THD	Total harmonic distortion
TORP	Total ossicular replacement prosthesis
VSB	Vibrant Soundbridge

accepted. In addition, computer models have been developed to simulate the sound transfer function (STF) under different conditions. The model simulations provide details of the complex vibration patterns and the data of the frequency specific cochlea input.

The AMEIs form the artificial part of the combined mechanical system. These devices were primarily developed for the healthy middle ear and the intact ossicular chain to replace conventional hearing aids in special cases such as external ear canal problems. Their use in chronic otitis media was not in the range of indications for implantable hearing devices for several medical and mechanical reasons. Colletti[1] was the first surgeon to place an AMEI on the stapes head and in the round window (RW) niche. Experiments on coupling implantable hearing aids together with passive middle ear prosthesis were performed during the same time period.[2] Consequently, the classical indication for implantable hearing devices was extended to chronic otitis media and reconstructed ossicular chain. The advantages are obvious. Although in cases of passive middle ear prosthesis, the tympanic membrane is the driving force for the reconstructed ossicular chain, after insertion of an AMEI, the power comes from the device itself. The tympanic membrane is no longer necessary for the sound transfer to the ossicular chain because, in many cases, insufficient function of the pathologically changed tympanic membrane seems to explain poor hearing results. AMEIs can also be considered to be a solution for dysfunction of the tympanic membrane in cases of middle ear effusion. However, apart from this advantage, there are many unanswered questions concerning AMEI application from the biomechanical point of view:

- Are there any differences in the mechanical characteristics of the currently available devices, and if so, how do they affect reconstruction?
- What is the best coupling site for an AMEI in the different middle ear situations?
- How can the device be coupled to the ossicular chain and what is the best direction of coupling?

This article does not intend to provide answers to all the questions but rather will attempt to summarize the current knowledge concerning the mechanical interaction between AMEIs and the normal or reconstructed middle ear. Some basic characteristics of the different AMEIs are provided in conjunction with the middle ear mechanics.

The interaction of AMEIs and middle ear and the influence of various boundary conditions are discussed in more detail and presented according to the different surgical situations.

BASICS OF SOUND TRANSFER OF THE MIDDLE EAR—PRESENT KNOWLEDGE

The normal middle ear is the reference system whose performance AMEIs have to reach and surpass. The intact middle ear consists of the tympanic membrane, the 3 ossicles (malleus, incus, stapes) with ligaments and joints, and the air-filled tympanic cavity. This mechanical system is designed to transfer the sound waves from the external ear canal into mechanical vibrations of the tympanic membrane and ossicular chain. The vibration of the stapes results at least in the traveling wave of the inner ear. Because of the impedance difference between air and fluid, the function of the middle ear can be considered to couple the sound energy of the air to the inner ear and match the impedance difference as well. This function is mainly performed by the hydraulic factor between the tympanic membrane and the stapes footplate. The large area (90 mm^2) of the tympanic membrane compared with the relatively small area of the stapes footplate (3 mm^2) creates the pressure amplification of about 22 dB around the resonant frequency of the middle ear (1 kHz).[3] Other factors in sound transmission, such as the catenary factor of the tympanic membrane or the lever ratio of the chain, are marginal.

This well-known common knowledge about middle ear function has been supplemented by new information in the past 20 years obtained from LDV measurements on temporal bones and calculations using finite element models (FEMs). Applying both these methods provided new insights into the vibration mode of the tympanic membrane and ossicular chain.[4–7]

Vibration Mode of the Tympanic Membrane

In the intact middle ear, the tympanic membrane is the driving force for the ossicular chain. The bridge between the membrane and the ossicular chain is the malleus handle. Calculations and experiments have shown that the vibration pattern is frequency-dependent. Although at frequencies less than 1 kHz all points of the tympanic membrane move in-phase (inward-outward motion of the entire membrane), the vibration pattern greater than 1 kHz becomes more and more complex. Between 1 and 4 kHz, lower-order modes predominate, with an example being a butterfly vibration pattern and other modes similar to those of microphone membranes. Greater than 4 kHz, the vibration pattern demonstrates multiple obviously independently moving spots of the tympanic membrane (**Fig. 1**). From new stroboscopic measurements, Rosowski and colleagues concluded that the vibration pattern in the highest frequency range results from an interaction of the modal motion with traveling waves at the surface of the membrane.[8,9]

Vibration Mode of the Ossicular Chain

The vibration pattern of the ossicular chain is dominated by the tympanic membrane movement. Because of the translational motion of the entire membrane, up to 1 kHz, the malleus and incus rotate around an axis between the short process of incus and the anterior mallear ligament (**Fig. 2**). The resulting movement of the stapes is piston-like. Above the first resonant frequency, the different modes of the tympanic membrane lead to a 3-dimensional vibration pattern of the chain. The rotational axis of the malleus and incus is shifted in a manner that is frequency-dependent to their upper part, the incudomalleolar joint and the incudostapedial joint become more mobile, and

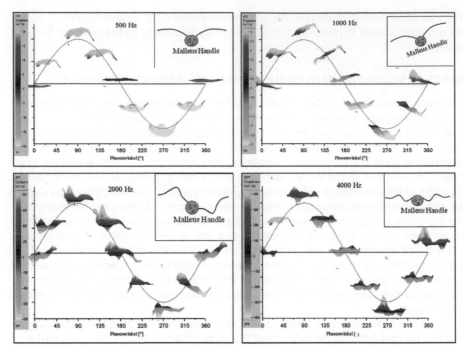

Fig. 1. Vibration mode of the tympanic membrane (TM). Displacements of the TM are displayed at different phases of one vibration cycle at 0.5, 1, 2, and 4 kHz.

the movement of the stapes becomes a combination of pistonlike and tilting movements as well as rotational components (**Fig. 3**).[10,11]

In the high-frequency range (greater than 4 kHz), the tilting movements can be in the same order of magnitude as the pistonlike movements. In animal experiments, it has been demonstrated that tilting movements also generate hearing sensations. After direct mechanical stimulation of the stapes with a transducer, compound action potentials were measured for tilting movements as well as for pistonlike movements, although the tilting movements were smaller (**Fig. 4**).[12,13]

Middle Ear Transfer Function

The middle ear transfer function (METF) has been calculated and measured in several models.[14–17] It describes, in general, the relation between the energy transmitted to the inner ear to the energy input in the external ear canal. Common definitions of the METF are (1) displacement of the stapes footplate related to the sound pressure at the tympanic membrane, (2) velocity of the stapes footplate related to the sound pressure at the tympanic membrane, or (3) sound pressure in the vestibulum related to the sound pressure at the tympanic membrane also named middle-ear pressure gain (GME). In this article, the first definition is usually meant when METF is used. **Fig. 5** shows the displacement of the stapes footplate related to the sound pressure at the tympanic membrane over frequency. The measurements were performed with LDV in temporal bones. The GME can be obtained from measurements of sound pressure in the vestibulum with hydrophones (**Fig. 6**). In the low-frequency range, GME increases with 6 dB per octave to a maximum of 23.5 dB at 1.2 kHz.[3] Above this frequency, the gain decreases with a slope of 6 dB per octave. The measurements

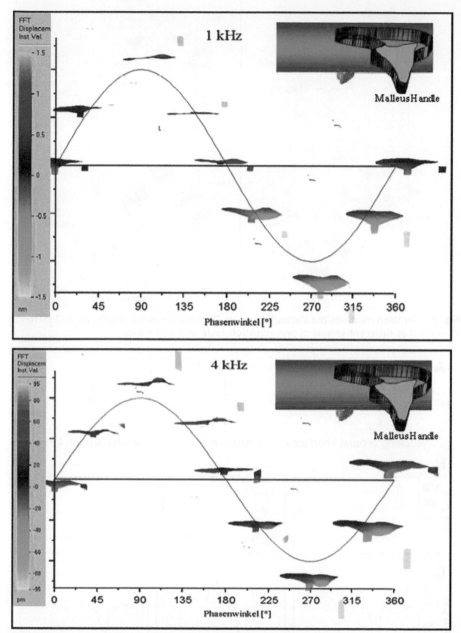

Fig. 2. Vibration mode of the malleus-incus complex. Displacements are displayed at different phases of one vibration cycle at 1 and 4 kHz.

demonstrated that the amplification of the middle ear is only about 22 dB in the frequency range between 0.5 and 1.5 kHz.

To characterize the interaction of AMEIs with the middle ear, observation of the vibration mode and data from STF are required. STF provides information on the overall energy transfer from the device to the middle ear. Vibration modes are useful for

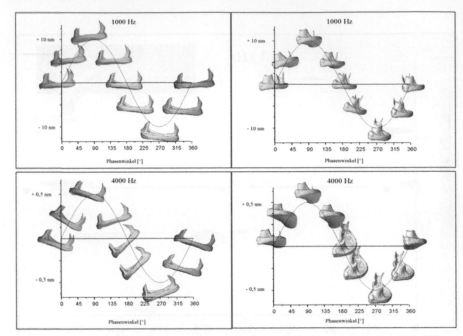

Fig. 3. Vibration mode of the stapes footplate. Displacements are displayed in 2 different views and at different phases of one vibration cycle at 1 and 4 kHz.

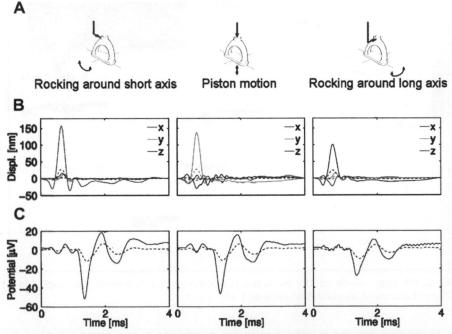

Fig. 4. Types of motion and compound action potentials (CAP). (*A*) Desired elementary motion; (*B*) measured motions; (*C*) measured CAP. Solid lines correspond to high-level excitation; dashed lines correspond to low-level excitation. (*From* Huber AM, Sequeira D, Breuninger C, et al. The effects of complex stapes motion on the response of the cochlea. Otol Neurotol 2008;29:1189; with permission.)

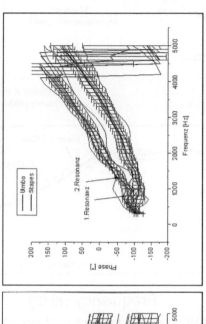

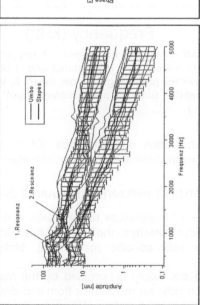

Fig. 5. Measured displacements at the umbo and the stapes footplate for sound pressure excitation at the tympanic membrane of 1 Pa (94 dB). The diagrams show the individual TFs of 10 temporal bone specimen and the mean *(red and blue line)* and standard deviation *(bars)*.

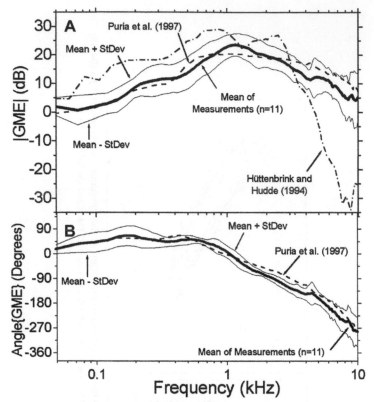

Fig. 6. Comparison of mean GME obtained in this study in 11 ears with mean GME reported by Puria and colleagues (1997) in 4 ears and Hüttenbrink and Hudde (1994) in 1 ear. (*A*) Shows magnitude and (*B*) shows the phase angle. (*From* Aibara R, Welsh JT, Puria S, et al. Human middle-ear sound transfer function and cochlear input impedance Hear Res 2001;152:106; with permission.)

optimizing coupling and stimulation characteristics. Of course, the mechanical behavior of the implantable hearing aid itself plays an important role.

MECHANICAL CHARACTERISTICS OF IMPLANTABLE HEARING DEVICES

A common characteristic of all implantable hearing aids is that the transducer is coupled to the ossicular chain or directly to the inner ear fluid. Consequently, implantable transducers have to fulfill specific mechanical, biological, and surgical requirements.

Mechanical requirements are mainly determined by the middle ear mechanics. Based on the knowledge of middle ear mechanics from experimental data and simulation models, the input impedance and motion of the ossicular chain are known. Thus, displacement and force characteristics for different points of the ossicular chain to which transducers may be coupled are provided. **Fig. 7**B shows the displacement of the stapes footplate (center point in direction of the footplate normal) at 1 Pa (equal to 94 dB sound pressure level (SPL)) sound pressure excitation at the tympanic membrane (green curve and scale on the left). The blue curve in **Fig. 7**A shows the required force acting on the stapes to produce the same displacement. That means that a

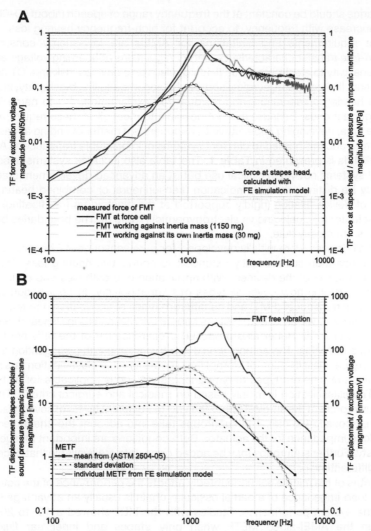

Fig. 7. (*A*) Measured force spectra of the FMT working against different impedance loads (*red, green, and black*). The force of the FMT is compared with the force necessary at the stapes head to generate stapes footplate displacements eq. to 94 dB SPL (1 Pa). The blue line (FE simulation model) shows the calculation with finite element model. (*B*) Measured free vibration amplitude of the FMT (at 50 mV excitation voltage) compared with the vibration amplitude at the stapes footplate (at 1-Pa sound pressure excitation at the tympanic membrane); mean and standard deviation of measurements of various research groups (ASTM) and calculated stapes footplate displacement for an individual middle ear.

transducer coupled to the stapes has to reach these values of force and displacement to produce a hearing sensation equivalent (eq.) to 94 dB SPL. Rosowski and colleagues[18] defined the eq. ear canal sound pressure as a measure to compare the performance of AMEI: the quotient of the electrovibrational transfer function (TF) (ie, the AMEI-aided METF) and the normal METF. It yields the eq. SPL that the transducer can generate in the middle ear for a certain driving voltage or current. The actuator performance should be constant at the frequency range of speech (about 90–6000 Hz) or even increase with frequency, to account for high-frequency hearing loss.

Further requirements and limitations for AMEIs are low-energy consumption, distortion-free transfer characteristics, safety regulations concerning voltage and current, insensitivity to electromagnetic fields of electronic devices, risk-free CT and MRI examination, limited space, surgical approach, biocompatibility, biostability, implantation with hearing preservation, and residue-free explantation,[19,20] to name just the most important ones. Because it is not possible to meet all of these requirements at the same time, developing implantable transducers is a matter of finding a reasonable compromise and this has led to different systems of implantable transducers. An overview of AMEIs is presented in **Table 1**. The table also includes systems used in the past and systems not yet in clinical use but at an advanced development stage. Devices may be distinguished by indication (sensorineural or combined hearing loss), the kind of device fixation (rigidly supported at the mastoid vs free floating), or the type of actuator (piezoelectric vs electrodynamic) (**Table 3**). The boundaries between the groups are mostly fluid.

Nearly all devices were initially developed for pure sensorineural hearing loss. The indication was then subsequently extended to conductive hearing loss. This trend boosted the usage of the devices. With application of prostheses and coupling elements, the systems now cover all types of tympanoplasty. In conjunction with the floating mass transducer (FMT) and its different types of application, the term "vibroplasty" is currently widely used.[2,21] At the Middle Ear Mechanics in Research and Otology meeting in 2006, Huber also proposed a classification of the different types of applications of AMEIs. The authors would like to implement this suggestion and propose a surgical classification of vibroplasty (**Table 2**). This classification is similar to the definition of different types of tympanoplasty[22] and is applicable for all types of AMEIs. The classification is mainly based on medical and surgical criteria. The main types thus represent the surgical approach and the different levels of severity and risks (infection, acoustic trauma). The subgroups take into account the attachment point and the load impedance for the actuator. Both conditions are important for successful vibroplasty. Further subgroups may be added once data are available that necessitate refined differentiation.

The status of the middle ear undoubtedly affects the performance of the actuator. A reduced load impedance of a partial ossicular chain is usually an advantage that improves the system performance. Studies with the MET showed a 10- to 20-dB increase in the AMEI-aided METF when only stapes and inner ear fluid were present.[23] With a partial ossicular chain, the required force of the actuator decreases, whereas the required displacement remains the same. An exception is direct cochlea fluid excitation, which might require greater displacements depending on the piston diameter (for details, see Mechanical aspects of type D vibroplasty). It will also be more difficult to use the direct acoustic cochlear stimulator (DACS) off-label (ie, to drive the ossicular chain), demanding greater force. The DACS is more attributed to the force-driven (ie, force-limited devices).

Many devices are rigidly supported with one end attached to a bony structure (cranium, tympanic cavity wall, ear canal wall). The other end is attached to the ossicular chain or the inner ear fluid. The sole exception of a free-floating actuator is the Vibrant Soundbridge (VSB)'s FMT that is only coupled to the ossicular chain. Electrodynamic actuators with separated coil and magnet are in between, because the coil is usually fixed in the ear canal and the magnet is attached to the ossicular chain. The rigidly supported transducers require more care for placement and the surgical procedure is usually more difficult. However, there is more space available in the mastoid than

Table 1
Overview of active middle ear implants

System	Company, Institution	Implantation Semi	Total	Actuator Electrodynamic	Piezoelectric	Coupling Umbo, TM	Malleus, Incus Body	Incus Long Process	Stapes	OW	RW	Cochlea	Published Studies Experimental	Clinical
Soundbridge	Med-El	x		x			x	x	Head, footplate	x	x	x	x	x
Esteem	Envoy Medical Corp.		x		x			x	Head				x	x
(MET), Carina	Otologics	(x)[a]	x	x			x	x	Head, footplate	x			x	x
C-DACS[b]	Cochlear	x		x							x	x	x	x
DACS-PI[b]	Sonova	x		x							x	x	x	x
Rion Device E-type	Japan	x			x				Head					x
TICA	Implex, Universität Tübingen, Germany		x		x		x	x					x	x
DDHS	Scundtec	x		x		x			Head					
SIMEHD	Cleveland, OH, USA	x		x				x					x (Animal)	
AMEI Tübingen	Universität Tübingen, Germany	x			x					x			x	x
Ear Lens	EarLens Corp., USA	x		x			x						x	x

[a] MET is semi-implantable, successor to Carina total implantable.
[b] Systems use the same actuator.
Data from Refs. 1,2,21,23,24,27,33–35,37–41,49,57,62–65,69–84

Table 2
Classification of vibroplasty (ie, middle ear reconstructions with active middle ear implants)

Vibroplasty	Description	Characteristics	Subtype	Coupling Location	AMEI
Type A	Coupling to the intact ossicular chain	Driving the whole and intact chain	A1	Tympanic membrane, malleus handle	DDHS, Ear lens
			A2	Incus body, malleus head	Soundbridge, Carina, SIMEHD
			A3	Incus long process	Soundbridge, Carina
			A4	Stapes footplate	(Carina)[a]
Type B	Coupling to interrupted/ reconstructed chain	Driving a part of the ossicular chain	B1	Incus body	TICA, Soundbridge
			B2	Incus long process, stapes head	Rion, TICA, Soundbridge, Carina, Esteem
			B3	Stapes footplate	Soundbridge, Carina
Type C	Membrane coupling to the inner ear	Driving the inner ear fluid via membrane	C1	RW	Soundbridge, Esteem, Carina, DACS, AMEI T.
			C2	Oval window with membrane	
			C3	Third window	Soundbridge
Type D	Inner ear fluid coupling	Driving the inner ear fluid directly	D1	Via RW	
			D2	Via oval niche	Soundbridge, DACS
			D3	Via third window	

[a] Possible but not used so far.

in the tympanic cavity, which allows for stronger transducers. The systems with separated coil and magnet can combine the advantages of easy placement and bigger coils and magnets. Their big drawback, that the performance heavily depends on the distance between coil and magnet, however, outweighs these advantages.

The devices can also be differentiated by the type of transducer: piezoelectric versus electrodynamic (electromagnetic), the latter with combined or separated coil and magnet. Depending on the specific design, piezoelectric transducers usually reach higher forces but are more limited in displacement. The opposite usually holds for electrodynamic transducers. If the operating range between the 2 idealized actuators, force-driven and displacement driven, is defined, nearly all current devices are within this range. In **Fig. 8**, the characteristics of the FMT can be seen as a typical example. At lower frequencies, the limited force of the FMT restricts the performance, whereas greater than 1 kHz, force and displacement are limiting factors. The force and displacement limits can be obtained from **Fig. 7**A, B, where forces and displacements in the middle ear are opposed to forces and displacements of the FMT.

Table 3
Characteristics of idealized and real actuators

Actuator type	Ideal displacement driven actuator	Real actuator	Ideal force driven actuator
Force characteristics	No limitation (ie, the actuator can generate more force than necessary)	Due to limitations in size, mass and energy usually a resonance characteristics with less force at low or high frequencies	The achievable force of the actuator limits the eq. SPL that the actuator can generate (in the whole frequency range)
Load impedance	Insensitive to the load impedance; actuator characteristics is independent from the attached structure	The achievable force and the frequency characteristics depend on the characteristics of the individual middle ear and the coupling point	Sensitive to the load impedance; the attached structure determines the actuator characteristics
Displacement characteristics		Usually limited displacement at low frequencies due to size and design limitations and safety considerations concerning excitation voltage	No limitation (ie, the displacement of the actuator in unloaded condition is larger than necessary)
Actuator examples	Stacked piezo actuator[26]	Most devices in **Table 1**	Electrodynamic actuator with separate coil and magnet (eg, EarLens[83])

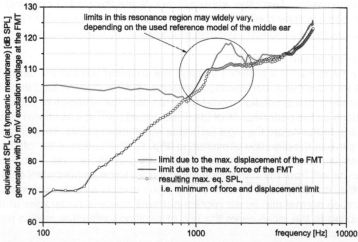

Fig. 8. Maximum eq. SPL of the FMT for 50 mV excitation voltage. The maximum eq. SPL is determined by the force limit (low-frequency range) and the displacement limit of the FMT.

Because of limitations in size, energy, tolerable voltage, and other boundary conditions, to date, it is not possible to achieve sufficient force and displacement over the entire frequency range. Therefore, transducers need to be designed to find an optimum in between. Javel and colleagues[24] showed the variation in performance for various designs of a piezoelectric bending transducer. Many actuators operate in resonance modes to minimize energy consumption. The resonance of the actuator is usually tuned to the first middle ear resonance at about 1 kHz and allows for high eq. SPL over a broad frequency range (0.9–6 kHz) with minimal energy consumption. It also provides actuator TFs with the same frequency characteristics as the METF (ie, a resonance around 1 kHz) (see **Fig. 7**B). This design is implemented in many electro-dynamic actuators (eg, VSB, DACS). Some piezoelectric actuators also use resonances, but mostly at higher frequencies to improve amplification for high-frequency hearing loss (eg, TICA with resonance around 7 kHz[25]). The TICA reached 130 dB eq. SPL at 10 kHz with only 0.2 mW energy consumption.[26] The resonance design of the actuators also leads to a performance that depends on load impedance and thus varies with individual middle ears and attachment points. For this reason, greater variation of AMEI performance than variation in METF should be expected. In principle, piezoelectric transducers may also be designed as stacked actuators with much higher force level, as Mills and colleagues[27] demonstrated. However, energy consumption then increases to about 70 mV.

SOUND TRANSFER OF THE MIDDLE EAR WITH ACTIVE MIDDLE EAR IMPLANTS
Coupling of Active Middle Ear Implants to the Intact Ossicular Chain: Type a Vibroplasty

Type A vibroplasty means provision of implantable hearing aids in the case of an intact ossicular chain (ie, the treatment of moderate sensorineural hearing loss). Most of the current devices were initially developed for this type of hearing loss. The performance of the devices is determined not only by the device itself but also by various boundary conditions on which the surgical procedure may have a bearing. The devices use different attachment points to the ossicular chain (eg, umbo, incus, or stapes), raising the question as to whether and how coupling positions and directions may influence actuator performance. Two other important points are the kind of coupling between transducer and ossicular chain and the possible pretension of the chain (annular ligament), because these conditions may also be controlled by the surgeon to a great extent.

Coupling position and direction
As already mentioned in a previous section, the coupling point at the ossicular chain influences the transducer performance because of differences in load impedance. A theoretic study with a simulation model demonstrated the influence of coupling points and directions on the performance of idealized actuators.[17] It was shown that the stapes head and footplate are the most favorable attachment points. These positions are also insensitive to the direction of excitation (**Fig. 9**). A direction of 60° off the longitudinal stapes axis reduced the achieved eq. SPL by only about 5 dB. Force-driven actuators can benefit from the impedance matching (ie, force amplification) of the middle ear when they are coupled to the umbo. The incus body is an unfavorable attachment point. Because normal middle ear motion patterns possess nodal lines at the incus body, coupling to the incus bears the risk of exciting ineffective motion patterns of the ossicular chain.

Experimental studies with real AMEIs support these theoretic findings. Devéze and colleagues[23] observed significantly better results (about 5–15 dB improvement) for the

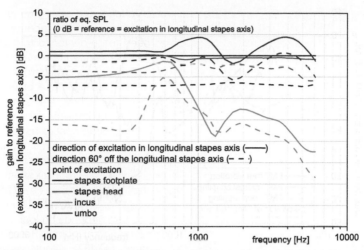

Fig. 9. Relative eq. SPL of an ideal force-driven actuator when coupled to different points of the ossicular chain. Directions of excitation were in the direction of the longitudinal stapes axis and at an angle of 60° to this axis. Results are based on simulations with an FE middle ear model. (*Data from* Bornitz M, Hardtke HJ, Zahnert T. Evaluation of implantable actuators by means of a middle ear simulation model. Hear Res 2010;263:145–51. http://dx.doi.org/10.1016/j.heares.2010.02.007.)

otologics device when AMEIs were coupled to the incus long process (near the stapes head) instead of the incus body.

Manufacturers whose devices use the incus as an attachment point (Esteem for sensor; MET, Carina, and TICA for actuator) are aware of the potential problems. They usually perform studies to find an optimal attachment point at the incus.[28] Studies have also shown that attachment at the incus may be as good as at the stapes. Mills and colleagues[27] placed a piezoelectric stack actuator in the attic region of the ear that drives the incus, obtaining eq. SPL of 90 to 130 dB at 1 to 6 kHz with 3.5 V_{rms} (root-mean-square voltage) driving voltage. Schraven and colleagues[29] attached the FMT to the short incus process and compared this position with the standard attachment at the long incus process. They observed on average about a 5-dB loss in AMEI-TF at the short incus process with standard deviation between 5 and −20 dB. Because of these large individual variations, it appears to be advisable to use some kind of intra-operative testing when coupling devices to the incus.

Coupling condition

Most studies use the terms "loose" and "tight" coupling to differentiate the coupling conditions. In the best case of tight coupling, perfect rigid coupling between transducer and ossicular chain can be assumed, which in reality only rarely occurs. Some actuators just touch the ossicular chain (eg, Otologics MET, Boulder, CO). A certain static preload to the actuator is needed to ensure a permanent contact. Other devices (eg, VSB) use crimping or clip mechanism for attachment. These mechanisms may reach nearly rigid coupling depending on the design, the surgical procedure, and skills of the surgeon. In most cases, however, there will be sliding at the interface for certain degrees of freedom or even changing contact (depending on frequency and excitation level). Loose coupling usually means the latter, where the transducer partly loses contact to the ossicle during 1 vibration cycle. Poor attachment is manifested by reduced TFs and increased harmonic distortion (**Fig. 10**).

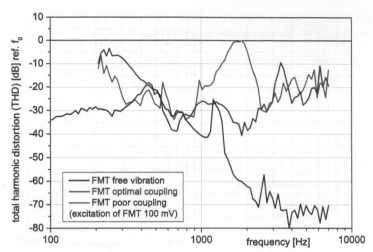

Fig. 10. THD of the FMT in free vibration and coupled to the incus long process in 2 different conditions (see **Fig. 11**). THD of 0 dB means the sum of the amplitudes of the higher harmonics is equal to the amplitude of the excitation frequency.

Crimping or clip mechanisms aim to provide rigid coupling. However, because of the spring-back of the material, elasticity crimping never provides real form closure. Thus, in reality, coupling is mostly achieved by adhesive forces and can be demonstrated with the FMT coupled to the incus long process (**Fig. 11**A, B). The FMT itself has a very linear vibration characteristic. Its total harmonic distortion (THD) is less than −20 dB (see **Fig. 10**, *black line*). This THD increases when the FMT is coupled to the ossicular chain, even if the FMT touches the stapes head and the attachment clip is tightly crimped to the incus long process (see **Fig. 10**, *blue line*). The reason is most likely an imperfect rigid coupling between transducer and ossicular chain. As a result, the contact between transducer and ossicle changes during one cycle of vibration. Similar relative movements were also shown for piston prostheses attached at the incus.[30] The THD increases further if the FMT is moved away from the stapes head (see **Fig. 10**, *red line*). Around 2 kHz, the harmonic distortions now

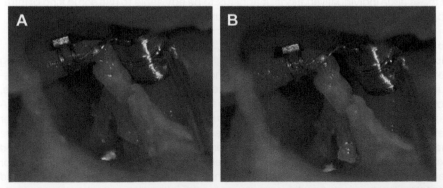

Fig. 11. (*A*) FMT coupled to the incus long process with optimal tight attachment. (*B*) FMT coupled to the incus long process without contact to the stapes head, resulting in poor attachment.

reach the same level as the excitation fundamental frequency. The middle ear can be excluded as a possible source, because it is a linear system, at least up to 100 dB SPL,[31] and the actuator performance is less than 90 dB eq. SPL at lower frequencies.

Snik and Cremers[32] used bone cement for additional fixation of the FMT and to ensure nearly rigid coupling conditions. They found a 10-dB better performance at 2 kHz compared with the control group with a crimped attachment clip alone. It was not reported whether the FMT also touched the stapes head; this may explain their large data variation. Lenarz and colleagues[33] also reported on better results with bone cement. These results support the theory that form closure of clip and crimp coupler alone does not ensure tight coupling. Additional adhesive forces between coupler and bone are required for tight coupling.

If the transducer is not directly coupled to the ossicles, but via an attachment clip (as in the second case, see **Fig. 11**B), then the stiffness of this attachment clip is also important. Wang and colleagues[5] used a simulation model to demonstrate that resonances of the attachment clips cause loss in the electrovibrational TF.

Contact problems arise from actuators that couple to the incus body or malleus head (eg, TICA, MET, Carina). Clip elements, which ensure better coupling at other points of the ossicular chain, cannot be used there. Just touching the ossicle with a small tip does not provide sufficient contact. The MET performed about 10 dB better if a clip coupler (MVP) was used compared with just touching the incus long process.[23] A disconnection in pulling direction may be prevented by pretension in the actuator attachment. However, this may cause excessive prestress (and thus stiffening) in the ossicular chain and mechanical overload of the actuator. These problems became evident when Otologics applied a new intraoperative loading instrumentation for the Carina system that assists in coupling the actuator.[34] The instrumentation optimizes the pretension in the actuator attachment. The performance of the AMEI dramatically improved by 10 to 20 dB with a new instrumentation, and variability of results was reduced. To ensure proper coupling of the actuator, some systems (eg, Esteem, TICA) always use surgical cement.[35,36]

Actuator-ossicular chain interference

Actuators coupled to the ossicular chain will always influence the normal METF. Contrary to conventional hearing aids, the devices cannot be simply removed in case of malfunction but require surgery, raising questions as to actuator-ossicular chain interactions in the case of inactive devices.

Actuators coupled to the ossicle without support to the surrounding bone (eg, the FMT) influence normal METF by their inertial mass. Experimental investigations concerning this issue remain inconsistent. Schraven and colleagues[29] did not find a significant effect of the passive FMT (coupled to the incus) on normal METF. A mean loss in TF of about 5 dB for frequencies greater than 3 kHz was observed with about 5 dB SD. Needham and colleagues[37] reported a 0- to 28-dB loss in METF at frequencies at or greater than 1 kHz if the FMT (about 30 mg) was coupled to the incus long process. The wide variability, however, indicates other boundary conditions as the source, such as different coupling conditions, because the selected coupling was not reliably reproducible (crimping at the incus process with no defined position of the FMT at or away from the stapes head). Another study with mass loading at the incus long process found changes of less than 5 dB for similar additional mass.[31] In this case, the mass was always glued to the ossicles.

Actuators supported at the surrounding bone and coupled to the ossicular chain (such as Carina, TICA) may block the movement of the ossicle because of the high actuator impedance. Actuator impedance is generally greater than middle ear impedance. A clinical study with the Carina system, however, did not show any significant shift in auditory thresholds after device implantation.[34] An experimental study with a stack piezo-actuator found less than 10-dB loss in METF.[27] The actuator was placed in the attic region and fixed with cement at both ends to the wall of the tympanic cavity and the incus, respectively. These results indicate that the actuator coupling is less ideally rigid than supposed, even with the use of cement.

The actuator-ossicular chain interference is not a one-way phenomenon, although the mechanical impedance of the actuator is greater than that of the middle ear. Coupling to the ossicular chain shifts the resonance of the actuator toward lower frequencies and reduces the actuator TF, especially at and above the actuator resonance. Quantitative data can only be found for the TICA.[25] Here, the resonance of the actuator changes from 10 kHz to around 7 kHz when coupled to the incus. This effect increases with decreasing mechanical impedance of the actuator. It is thus usually greater for electrodynamic actuators than for piezoelectric actuators. The changes in mechanical characteristics of the actuator, of course, also induce changes in the electrical characteristics of the actuator. These changes in electrical impedance of the actuator can be used to control the coupling to the ossicular chain.[34] For this application, electrodynamic actuators are ahead of piezoelectric types because of the usually lower mechanical impedance of electrodynamic actuators. Coupling to the ossicular chain induces bigger changes in the electrical impedance and changes in actuator coupling are easier to detect.

Coupling of Active Middle Ear Implants to Remnants of the Ossicular Chain: Type B Vibroplasty (B2/B3)

Position: experimental data for coupling of active middle ear implants to the stapes (head/footplate)

In addition to coupling to the intact ossicular chain, most AMEIs can also be attached to the stapes or its footplate. This possibility additionally allows for their use in the chronically disabled middle ear and is therefore a considerable expansion over devices designed for the intact ossicular chain alone.

A direct coupling of the FMT to the stapes head (fixed with bone cement) on one side and the tympanic membrane in the normal anatomic position on the other side (with cartilage slice interposition) is possible and results in comparable amplification results as for the "classical" coupling site on the long process of the incus.[38] Nevertheless, the use of additional couplers to secure the FMT-ossicle interface has become accepted. Like reconstructions with passive prostheses, a coupling to the stapes head (partial ossicular replacement prosthesis [V-PORP]) or to the stapes footplate (total ossicular replacement prostheses [V-TORP]) in the case of an absent superstructure is possible. Most experimental and simulation data are available for the FMT (Med-El, Innsbruck, Austria). In addition to the previously described use in the intact ossicular chain (see Coupling of AMEIs to the intact ossicular chain, type A vibroplasty), the FMT can be attached to couplers and thereby coupled to the stapes.

Type B2 vibroplasty: coupling to the stapes head

Two different coupling devices are available that aim for firm and stable FMT placement on the stapes head. The Bell-Vibroplasty is assembled from a titanium PORP (Bell Tübingen; Kurz, Dusslingen, Germany). In this case, the FMT and the prosthesis strut show a parallel alignment.[2] Another system uses the Dresden Clip mechanism (Kurz) or the Bell system for a serial alignment of the FMT on top of the stapes head.[39] Both the parallel and the serial alignment provide transmission properties like the original passive prostheses if the reconstruction supplies a contact to the (reconstructed) tympanic membrane and the FMT is not activated.

Temporal bone experiments using the parallel V-PORP assembly document a maximal vibration eq. to an SPL of 108 to 125 dB at the tympanic membrane when driving the FMT with a 100-mV input.[2] At the same coupling site (stapes head), Shimizu and colleagues[40] measured an SPL eq. of 112 to 118 SPL. These results are approximately 10 dB lower than 3 kHz and 10 dB higher at frequencies greater than 6 kHz when using a serial FMT-V-PORP assembly. The differences between these studies are not clear but can be caused by the FMT-coupler assembly (parallel/serial), the measuring system and stimulation, the annular ligament pretension, or the use of a third window in the study by Shimizu and colleagues.

The actuators of the other AMEIs directly drive the stapes or its footplate without any combination with a conventional passive middle ear prosthesis. Hence, a passive sound transmission with the inactivated device is not given. The piezoelectric Esteem driver experimentally reaches stapes displacements eq. to 100 to 110 dB SPL with 1-V pp stimulus, extendible up to 120 to 130 dB SPL with a 10-V stimulus.[28] For the MET of the Carina system (second-generation Middle Ear Transducer, Otologics), experimental data for a direct stapes stimulation with a Bell tip have shown the best amplification results. Because of the load reduction after removal of the malleus and incus, the mean gain was up to 22 dB.[23] Even though the system can be equipped with different tip modifications for direct footplate stimulation, no experimental data are available for that specific condition.

Type B3 vibroplasty: coupling to the stapes footplate

As mentioned above, in the case of an absent stapes superstructure, direct coupling of the actuator to the stapes footplate is necessary. For this case also, the FMT can be assembled with commercial passive V-TORP in a parallel or serial manner. For serial alignment of the FMT and the prosthesis device, a titanium FMT-Clipholder (Kurz) is used, and the strut is positioned on the center of the footplate.

Temporal bone experiments showed a 20-dB gain in the middle and high frequencies with the activated FMT (50-mV) compared with the intact ossicular chain (with 95-dB acoustic stimulation).[21] Although no experimental data are available for the parallel FMT-TORP assembly, which is already in clinical use,[41] an eq. amplification can be assumed. A serial V-PORP measurement produced a response of 112 to 118 dB SPL (1.0–8.0 kHz, 316 mV FMT input), with a slightly inferior performance in the frequencies greater than 5 kHz.[40] When comparing the V-PORP with the V-TORP reconstruction in the same study, an up to 9 dB SPL better performance for the V-PORP at frequencies greater than 2 kHz was found.

For all other AMEIs, no experimental data for a direct footplate coupling are available, although some of them can be used in this fashion.

Positioning: influence of force axis between actuator and stapes

The complex physiologic vibration patterns of the ossicular chain, especially rocking and tilting movements of the stapes, are only partly reproducible with mechanical stimulation by an actuator. Even if mainly pistonlike movements are generated by an actuator, the angle between the stapes' z-axis and the main axis of the driver's force influences the quality of the mechanical stimulation.

In FEM simulations, an angle deviation of 20 to 60° between the stapes' z-axis and the actuator's force axis causes a decrease of 3 to 10 dB. This effect also depends on the coupling site of the actuator with a generally higher transmission decrease if the actuator is coupled to the stapes' footplate (**Fig. 12**).[17]

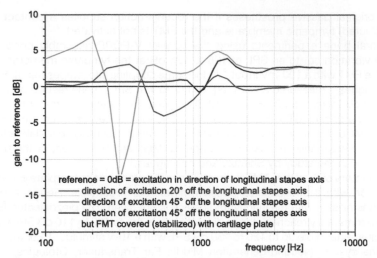

Fig. 12. Relative eq. SPL of an ideal force-driven actuator when coupled to the stapes head. The incus had been removed. Directions of excitation were in the direction of the longitudinal stapes axis and at an angle of 20° to 45° to this axis. Results are based on simulations with an FE middle ear model. (*Data from* Bornitz M, Hardtke HJ, Zahnert T. Evaluation of implantable actuators by means of a middle ear simulation model. Hear Res 2010;263:145–51. http://dx.doi.org/10.1016/j.heares.2010.02.007.)

Tension: influence of cartilage shielding and annular ligament prestress

The function of AMEIs in chronic otitis with poor middle ear ventilation, a tympano-sclerotic middle ear mucosa, middle ear effusion, and stable cartilage reconstruction of the tympanic membrane was experimentally investigated for the FMT. Analogously to intact ossicular chain (see Coupling of AMEIs to the intact ossicular chain, type A vibroplasty), these conditions can lead to an annular ligament prestress and its consecutive stiffening, resulting in a reduced TF.

When coupling the FMT (50 mV) to the stapes (V-TORP) without any fixation on the opposite side (tympanic membrane), up to 20 dB transfer loss can be observed.[42] Similar to passive prosthesis reconstructions, this is due to loose coupling conditions between the prosthesis and the stapes and/or the (reconstructed) tympanic membrane. When using AMEIs, STF decrease is caused by a contact loss of the AMEI and the ossicle during a vibration cycle. When the FMT is covered with cartilage, the pistonlike movements along the z-axis are intensified, because the vibrations in the other degrees of freedom are assumed to be suppressed. Simultaneously, the connection between the FMT-coupler and the stapes is stabilized by preventing a clearance in the interface. Experimentally, increasing the cartilage pressure on the V-TORP can simulate poor middle ear aeration and scar tissue formation, resulting in a stepwise reduction in the TF of up to 25 dB. This effect is predominantly seen in the frequencies less than 4 kHz.[42]

To investigate the isolated effect of an annular ligament pretension, the authors measured the TF with respect to the footplate displacement. A 67-μm footplate displacement toward the vestibule stiffened the annular ligament by ×15 and reduced the TF by 20 dB in the low-frequency and mid-frequency range (**Fig. 13**). This footplate displacement stresses the importance that, just as in the use of passive prostheses, in AMEIs the pretension for the annular ligament should be as low as possible.

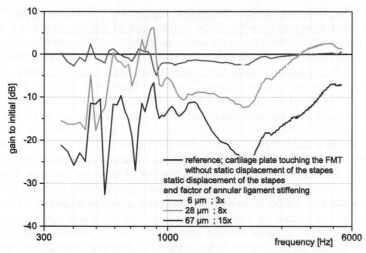

Fig. 13. Decrease in eq. SPL of the FMT coupled to the stapes head because of stiffening of the annular ligament. The FMT was covered with a cartilage plate, which was stepwise moved toward the stapes. At the reference condition (=0 dB), the cartilage plate just touches the FMT without static displacement of the stapes.

Interestingly, the effect of a middle ear effusion simulated by filling the oval niche around the V-TORP (50-mV FMT stimulation) was comparably small. The TF was reduced by only 5 dB in the frequency range from 0.5 to 2.0 kHz.[42]

For the other AMEIs, experimental or simulation data on the influence of pathologic middle ear conditions and a direct coupling to the stapes head or its footplate are not available.

Coupling of Active Middle Ear Implants to the Round Window: Type C Vibroplasty

Colletti and colleagues[1] described the VSB coupling at the RW in patients with destroyed stapes or middle ear malformation. Since this publication, coupling at the RW has become an increasingly common alternative for coupling the VSB. Good hearing results after RW-coupling[1,43–49] also legitimize this method in cases of intact chain, present stapes, or otosclerosis. During surgery, it is sometimes difficult to expose the round window membrane (RWM). It depends on the bony structures around the window and the position of the membrane outside the microscopic view axis. For this reason, the only current implantable hearing device for RW coupling appears to be the VSB. On the other hand, Tringali and colleagues[50] described the coupling of the Middle Ear Transducer (Otologics LLC) with a ball tip onto the RW.

Pau and Just[51] reported a case of coupling the FMT onto a third window by preserving the endothelial tissue, which is another possibility for type C vibroplasty that is comparable to RW-coupling. The coupling actuator to oval niche after opening the inner ear and reclosing with soft tissue membrane should also be included in this vibroplasty type. Devéze and colleagues[52] observed in such a manner of stimulation around 4 dB better performance gains than directly driven inner ear fluid. The RW-coupling is the most common type C vibroplasty.

Round window conditions

It seems that the RW is a perfect gate to reach the inner ear. There is only a thin membrane between the fluid of the inner ear and the aerated middle ear. The RWM presents the only nonosseous wall of the labyrinth. It has 3 distinct layers: the tympanic layer, the intermediate connective tissue, and the internal layer.[53] Sound takes the same direction from the base to the apex of the cochlea, but it starts in the scala tympani rather than the scala vestibuli. With human temporal bone measurement and direct comparison between RW and stapes coupling, however, Shimizu and colleagues[40] found better results with stapes coupling. Does this mean that RW coupling is always the second choice? The mean transverse diameter of the RWM was 1.65 mm in the study conducted by Su and colleagues.[54] The mean width of the RW niche was 1.66 mm and the mean depth was 1.34 mm, independent of age. The diameter of the FMT is 1.8 mm and the length 2.3 mm (**Fig. 14**). Because of the cable, the length is divided into 3 parts, 0.9 at both ends and 0.5 at the cable entrance. It therefore appears that the FMT is not perfectly suited for use of the RW gate. Furthermore, exposing the RWM increases the risk of inner ear damage. Comparing the 2 different possibilities of inner ear stimulation, normal forward sound stimulation and reverse RW stimulation, in reverse stimulation, the nondriven end of the cochlea is terminated by the middle ear output impedance. Nakajima and colleagues[55] found higher acoustic impedance for reverse stimulation. This impedance depends on the situation of middle ear structures. In the case of a destroyed stapes suprastructure and normal annular ligament, the impedance is lower than in the case of a fixed footplate or intact ossicular chain.

Position
AMEIs, except for the VSB-FMT, have to be fixed in the mastoid. Therefore, they have only a small amount of variability in positioning at the RW. The VSB-FMT is the only AMEI described for this type of use in patients. Because of the small size of the FMT, it offers a range of options for placing it at the RW. In general, however, the FMT is not the right size for implantation in the RW niche. It is necessary to widen the bony niche or to use a coupling material such as soft tissue or RW coupler for bridging. The RW coupler helps to find an effective position with centering the movement near the middle of RW, on the one hand, but on the other hand, it enlarges the diameter of the FMT (**Fig. 15**). Arnold and colleagues[56] investigated 5 different position conditions of the FMT (**Fig. 16**) and compared it to a bone-anchored hearing aid. They

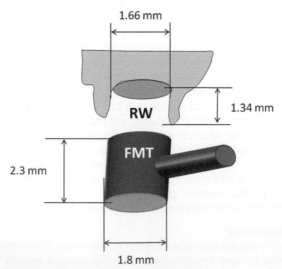

Fig. 14. Median size of the RW compared with FMT dimensions.

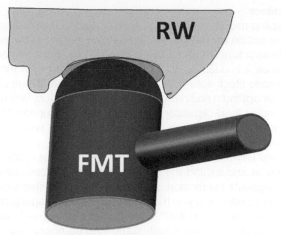

Fig. 15. Improved contact using FMT with RW-coupler.

measured displacements at the stapes and promontory if the FMT is placed directly at the RWM, with a soft tissue underlay or overlay, parallel to the RWM, fixed in the RW niche and at the promontory. The orientation and method of attachment substantially influence vibratory energy transfer to the cochlea by up to 40 dB. To achieve the best efficiency of labor, the FMT movement axis has to be in orthogonal projection to the RWM plane and must not contact bony structures. It was demonstrated that the VSB-FMT is not suitable as an implantable bone conduction hearing aid. Installing a brace between FMT and the hypotympanic wall increases the coupling to the RW[57] and stabilizes the FMT.

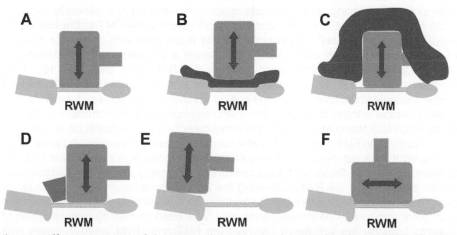

Fig. 16. Different positions of the FMT in the RW niche: (*A*) FMT directly coupled to the RW in orthogonal position, (*B*) orthogonal position with soft tissue underlay, (*C*) orthogonal position, like position "A" with soft tissue overlay, (*D*) tide fixed orthogonal position, (*E*) external position fixed at basal turn of cochlea, (*F*) parallel position. (*Adapted from* Arnold A, et al. The floating mass transducer at the round window: direct transmission or bone conduction? Hear Res 2010;263:122. http://dx.doi.org/10.1016/j.heares.2009.12.019; with permission.)

Tension and resistance

Pretension in coupling middle ear prostheses may lead to less dislocation and better contact. In passive middle ear prostheses, pretension increases the air bone gap. The RWM is a soft thin structure stabilized by collagen fibers. Schraven and colleagues[58] investigated pretension in coupling on RWM with a 0.5-mm cylindrical metal tip and driven by piezoelectric stack actuator. They suggested that 90-μm pretension of the RWM is essential for optimum and reproducible RW stimulation. Ishii and colleagues[59] observed an ascending load-displacement curve, and the rupture load was 564 mN with displacement of 122 μm. Force and displacement of working AMEIs are not known to the authors at present.

In coupling on the RWM, different findings for resistance are possible because of deviating situations at and behind the stapes footplate. Piezoelectric AMEIs deliver enough power to negotiate the tension. Electromechanical systems exhibit characteristic impedance curves depending on the mass damping and spring rate in the biological surroundings and the system itself. Tringali and colleagues[50] found a negligible difference in acoustic stapes velocity with static load compared with unloaded measurements. Arnold and colleagues[60] also did not observe any significant effect on energy transfer after interruption of the ossicular chain.

Contact

If a well-controlled mechanical contact of an inflexible actuator to the RWM is ensured, the resultant stimulation of the cochlea will be reproducible and have functionally relevant magnitude.[58] The coupling efficiency correlates directly with the amount of contact area between actuator and RWM.[61] The RW niche contains the RWM, and the bony frame is composed of the outer wall of the basal turn, the crista fenestra, the anteroinferior overhang, and the posterosuperior overhang. All of these structures may be contact areas for the AMEI. Because of the anteroinferior overhang and the posterosuperior overhang, intraoperative control of contact is impossible. As a result of this, and to adapt the size of the RW niche to the FMT, the anteroinferior overhang and the posterosuperior overhang are generally reduced while a VSB is implanted in this location. When coupling the FMT in the RW niche, Nakajima and colleagues[57] found better results in coupling with using 1 or 2 layers of soft tissue compared with a bare FMT. Arnold and colleagues[60] investigated 6 different possibilities for FMT positioning in the RW niche (see **Fig. 16**). They measured the FMT in parallel position with poor energy transfer and FMT oriented perpendicularly to the RWM with good energy transfer in the cochlea. If they included underlay tissue in these situations, they found an improved energy transfer to the cochlea. In clinical observation, Rajan and colleagues[61] observed better hearing results after coupling the FMT directly at the RW rather than using underlay soft tissue. They described it as a dampening of the vibrations due to the high compliance and low stiffness of the soft tissue with subsequent loss of energy across the distance between the FMT and the RWM. Covering the FMT with cartilage and soft tissue, as performed in their study, was intended to minimize the damping effect. This deviation from other temporal bone investigations may have been caused by their selection of patients because the soft tissue between the FMT and RWM, used in cases with mismatch between RWM and FMT diameter, should increase the coupling. However, in these patients, RW bony barrier problems may also have existed (**Fig. 17**). It therefore appears that the quality of contact to the RWM is one of the most important factors of energy transfer. The RW coupler should optimize the contact between FMT and RWM. The spherical surface of this device can adapt the contact area to the RWM size.

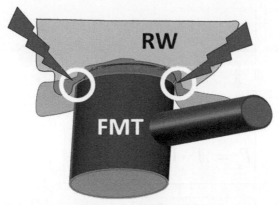

Fig. 17. FMT in orthogonal position with soft tissue underlay and suspected bone contact (*white circle* = contact area).

Tringali and colleagues[50] stimulated the RWM with 2 different ball tip diameters (0.5 and 1 mm). They drove the RW before and after drilling the bony rim. In this investigation, niche drilling increased the measured mean peak stapes velocities. Consequently, the bony surroundings of the RW niche present an obstacle in sound transmission when using AMEIs. The relations of size from tip and membrane diameter may exclude the contact between tip and bony frame of the membrane. Otherwise, the angle from tip movement direction and the membrane surface plane, especially before drilling, may lead to less membrane contact of the tip. The higher increase in measured mean peak stapes velocities while using the smaller tip supports this assumption. The tip diameter becomes relevant at higher frequencies of more than 4 kHz. At these frequencies, the 0.5-mm tip was more effective than the 1.0-mm diameter tip.

Mechanical Aspects of Type D Vibroplasty

Type D vibroplasty is defined as the direct coupling of an AMEI to the inner ear fluid. For this approach, the oval window (after stapedectomy or stapedotomy), the RW (after perforation), or a third window in the promontory can be used for this aim. The mechanical advantage involves the bridging of the impedance of the annular ligament. From stapesplasty, it is known that a small piston with a diameter of only 0.4 to 0.6 mm can bring about the same hearing results as the intact stapes; this is possible because if the annular ligament is intact, the volume displacement of the stapes is similar to the volume displacement of the stapes piston. Because of the missing impedance of the annular ligament, the stapes pistons move more deeply into the inner ear than the stapes itself (**Fig. 18**). Consequently, the volume displacement is similar in a frequency-dependent manner.

All of the problems of abnormal high annular ligament impedance can be resolved by coupling active or passive implants to the cochlear fluid. From the mechanical point of view, transferred energy depends on the vibration magnitude of the transducer and the diameter of the coupler. Concerning the diameter of the coupler, the same mechanical principle can be assumed as in stapesplasty: The bigger the diameter of the piston, the better the sound transfer to the cochlea (**Fig. 19**). Of course, this effect is also frequency-dependent. In the low-frequency range, sound transfer is in relation to the piston diameter. At higher frequencies, damping by the inner ear fluid can reduce the effect. The relation between piston diameter and STF is difficult to measure in temporal bones. Therefore, in addition to clinical data, calculations have been used to demonstrate the effect.[62]

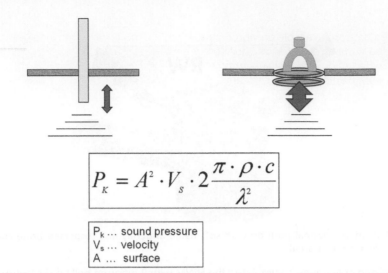

$$P_{K} = A^{2} \cdot V_{s} \cdot 2 \frac{\pi \cdot \rho \cdot c}{\lambda^{2}}$$

P_k ... sound pressure
V_s ... velocity
A ... surface

Fig. 18. Influence of the piston diameter to the sound transfer of the inner ear fluid. Both piston and stapes demonstrate similar volume displacements because the piston vibrates deeper into the inner ear fluid compared with the stapes.

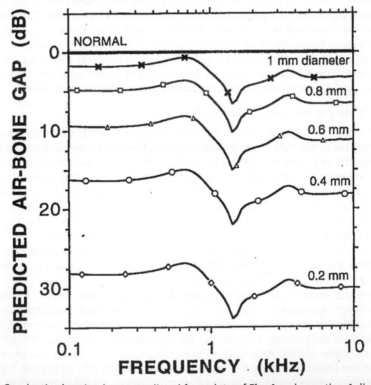

Fig. 19. Conductive hearing losses predicted from data of **Fig. 4** and equation 1 displayed in the style of a clinical audiogram. The air-bone gap in the normal ear is 0 dB. The air-bone gaps predicted for circular pistons of various diameters indicate progressive increase in the gap as the piston diameter decreases to less than 1 mm. (*From* Rosowski JJ, Merchant SN. Mechanical and acoustic analysis of middle ear reconstruction. Am J Otol 1995;16:491; with permission.)

Limited data are available on vibroplasty with direct coupling to the inner ear due to the limited number of patients who are suitable for this procedure. In the case of a contaminated middle ear cavity (chronic otitis media), every opening has a high risk of inner ear infection leading to hearing loss. Häusler and colleagues[63] first operated on 4 patients with otosclerosis using a new implantable hearing system, the DACS. The hearing threshold of the implanted ears before implantation ranged from 78 to 101 dB (air conduction, pure tone average, 0.5–4 kHz) with air-bone gaps of 33 to 44 dB in the same frequency range. Postoperatively, substantial improvements in sound field thresholds, speech intelligibility as well as in the subjective assessment of everyday situations were found in all patients. Two years after the implantations, monosyllabic word recognition scores in quiet at 75 dB improved by 45% to 100% points when using the DACS. The design of the DACS actuator and the acoustic characteristics were described in extent by Bernhard and colleagues.[64] The DACS System had also been investigated in temporal bones. The maximum gain (eq. SPL for an applied voltage of 0.3 V) in reconstruction with a DACS PI was excellent (>110 dB) up to the resonant frequency of 1.5 kHz, and greater than 90 dB for the higher frequencies. A self-crimping prosthesis was recommended for the use with the DACS PI System.[65] Lenarz and colleagues[66] introduced a clinical multicenter study of 15 patients with severe to profound mixed hearing loss because of otosclerosis with the CODACS System and found a mean sound field threshold (0.25–8 kHz) improvement of 48 dB. In addition to the DACS, the VSB is suitable for otosclerosis surgery as described by Dumon.[67] In cases of mixed hearing loss, the transducer was coupled conventionally to the long process of the incus in combination with a piston.[67,68] The technique (Power stapes) was also used in patients with osteogenesis imperfecta.[69] However, because of the inner ear infection risk, it cannot be recommended in all cases of chronic otitis media. The hearing gain was at the same level as for RWM coupling. Schwab and colleagues[70] presented a compromise to reduce the risk of infection. After resecting the footplate, they closed the oval niche with perichondrium. The transducer was coupled directly to the new membrane. However, all of the patients in the study had intact tympanic membranes and ventilated middle ear cavities. It is not known whether the impedance of the perichondrium used was less than the impedance of the annular ligament. Apart from coupling of a transducer to the vestibulum, the cochlea can also be reached through the RW niche or through a third window. These considerations are only theoretic, however, because the RW niche is narrow and difficult for a piston coupler to reach. The third window coupling was published in a clinical case of obliterative tympanosclerosis by Pau and Just.[51] The FMT was gently pushed into the perichondrium-coated cochlear window without any damage to the inner ear. The audiologic results were comparable with the conventional coupling of the FMT on the RW niche.

SUMMARY

The various AMEIs, combined with different middle ear situations, give rise to a wide range of different reconstructions. To structure the middle ear reconstructions with AMEIs, a classification was used based on medical and surgical criteria. The designation vibroplasty can be used for all types of AMEIs in the middle ear. It can be divided into 4 types (A–D), characterized by coupling the AMEI to the intact ossicular chain (A), to the interrupted or partial chain (B), to inner ear fluid via a membrane (C), and to inner ear fluid directly (D). The success of a vibroplasty depends on the AMEI performance and different boundary conditions of the vibroplasty types. The AMEI-aided METF depends on attachment point, direction, and condition. In principle, stapes head and footplate seem to be the most favorable attachment points. Coupling elements may help to achieve good (rigid) coupling between actuator and ossicular chain, although only glue and cement seem to ensure this condition. In the case of type B–C vibroplasty and the use of the FMT, it is advisable to use cartilage to stabilize the reconstruction and to optimize AMEI coupling. Pretension of the annular ligament due to large contact pressure with the AMEI can considerably decrease the TF, especially in type B vibroplasty. The RW coupling is the most common type C vibroplasty. Different investigations report good hearing results after RW-coupling. Temporal bone experiments show best STF if the FMT movement axis is in orthogonal projection to the RWM plane. The most important factor for energy transfer to the inner ear at the RW is the quality of contact between RWM and AMEI. This contact can be improved with coupler elements. The direct coupling to inner ear fluid should only be used in cases of noncontaminated middle ears. The advantage of type D vibroplasty is the bypass of the impedance of the stapes and annular ligament. There are currently very few clinical studies or temporal bone experiments concerning this type of vibroplasty.

REFERENCES

1. Colletti V, Soli SD, Carner M, et al. Treatment of mixed hearing losses via implantation of a vibratory transducer on the round window. Int J Audiol 2006;45:600–8. http://dx.doi.org/10.1080/14992020600840903.
2. Huber AM, Ball GR, Veraguth D, et al. A new implantable middle ear hearing device for mixed hearing loss: a feasibility study in human temporal bones. Otol Neurotol 2006;27:1104–9. http://dx.doi.org/10.1097/01.mao.0000244352. 49824.e6.
3. Aibara R, Welsh JT, Puria S, et al. Human middle-ear sound transfer function and cochlear input impedance. Hear Res 2001;152:100–9.
4. Zhang X, Gan RZ. A comprehensive model of human ear for analysis of implantable hearing devices. IEEE Trans Biomed Eng 2011;58:3024–7. http://dx.doi.org/10.1109/TBME.2011.2159714.
5. Wang X, Hu Y, Wang Z, et al. Finite element analysis of the coupling between ossicular chain and mass loading for evaluation of implantable hearing device. Hear Res 2011;280:48–57. http://dx.doi.org/10.1016/j.heares.2011.04.012.
6. Decraemer WF, Khanna SM, Gyo K, et al. Measurement, visualization and quantitative analysis of complete three-dimensional kinematical data sets of human and cat middle ear. In: Gyo K, Wada H, Hato N, et al, editors. Middle ear mechanics in research and otology. Singapore: World Scientific; 2004. p. 3–10.
7. Cheng JT, Aarnisalo AA, Harrington E, et al. Motion of the surface of the human tympanic membrane measured with stroboscopic holography. Hear Res 2010; 263:66–77. http://dx.doi.org/10.1016/j.heares.2009.12.024.
8. Cheng JT, Hamade M, Merchant SN, et al. Wave motion on the surface of the human tympanic membrane: holographic measurement and modeling analysis. J Acoust Soc Am 2013;133:918–37. http://dx.doi.org/10.1121/1.4773263.
9. Rosowski JJ, Cheng JT, Merchant SN, et al. New data on the motion of the normal and reconstructed tympanic membrane. Otol Neurotol 2011;32: 1559–67. http://dx.doi.org/10.1097/MAO.0b013e31822e94f3.
10. Huber AM, Eiber A. Vibration properties of the ossicle and cochlea and their importance for our hearing system. HNO 2011;59:255–60. http://dx.doi.org/10. 1007/s00106-011-2271-6.
11. Zahnert T. Laser in der Ohrforschung. Laryngorhinootologie 2003;82(Suppl 1): 157–80.

12. Huber AM, Sequeira D, Breuninger C, et al. The effects of complex stapes motion on the response of the cochlea. Otol Neurotol 2008;29(8):1187–92. http://dx.doi.org/10.1097/MAO.0b013e31817ef49b.

13. Eiber A, Huber AM, Lauxmann M, et al. Contribution of complex stapes motion to cochlea activation. Hear Res 2012;284:82–92. http://dx.doi.org/10.1016/j.heares.2011.11.008.

14. Nishihara S, Aritomo H, Goode RL. Effect of changes in mass on middle ear function. Otolaryngol Head Neck Surg 1993;109:899–910.

15. Voss SE, Rosowski JJ, Merchant SN, et al. Acoustic responses of the human middle ear. Hear Res 2000;150:43–69.

16. Kelly DJ, Prendergast PJ, Blayney AW. The effect of prosthesis design on vibration of the reconstructed ossicular chain: a comparative finite element analysis of four prostheses. Otol Neurotol 2003;24:11–9.

17. Bornitz M, Hardtke HJ, Zahnert T. Evaluation of implantable actuators by means of a middle ear simulation model. Hear Res 2010;263:145–51. http://dx.doi.org/10.1016/j.heares.2010.02.007.

18. Rosowski JJ, Chien W, Ravicz ME, et al. Testing a method for quantifying the output of implantable middle ear hearing devices. Audiol Neurootol 2007;12:265–76. http://dx.doi.org/10.1159/000101474.

19. Leysieffer H. Principle requirements for an electromechanical transducer for implantable hearing aids in inner ear hearing loss. I: technical and audiologic aspects. HNO 1997;45:775–86.

20. Zenner HP. Principle requirements of an electromechanical transducer for implantable hearing aids in inner hearing hearing loss. II: clinical aspects. HNO 1997;45(10):787–91.

21. Hüttenbrink KB, Zahnert T, Bornitz M, et al. TORP-vibroplasty: a new alternative for the chronically disabled middle ear. Otol Neurotol 2008;29:965–71. http://dx.doi.org/10.1097/MAO.0b013e318185fad8.

22. WULLSTEIN H. Theory and practice of tympanoplasty. Laryngoscope 1956;66:1076–93. http://dx.doi.org/10.1288/00005537-195608000-00008.

23. Devèze A, Koka K, Tringali S, et al. Techniques to improve the efficiency of a middle ear implant: effect of different methods of coupling to the ossicular chain. Otol Neurotol 2013;34:158–66. http://dx.doi.org/10.1097/MAO.0b013e3182785261.

24. Javel E, Grant IL, Kroll K. In Vivo Characterization of Piezoelectric Transducers for Implantable Hearing Aids. Otol Neurotol 2003;24:784–95.

25. Leysieffer H, Baumann JW, Müller G, et al. An implantable piezoelectric hearing aid transducer for inner ear deafness. II: clinical implant. HNO 1997;45:801–15.

26. Leysieffer H, Baumann JW, Müller G, et al. An implantable piezoelectric hearing aid transducer for inner ear hearing loss. I: development of a prototype. HNO 1997;45:792–800.

27. Mills RP, Wang ZG, Abel EW. In vitro study of a multi-layer piezoelectric crystal attic hearing implant. J Laryngol Otol 2001;115:359–62.

28. Kroll K, Grant IL, Javel E. The envoy totally implantable hearing system, St. Croix Medical. Trends Amplif 2002;6:73–80.

29. Schraven SP, Dalhoff E, Wildenstein D, et al. Alternative fixation of an active middle ear implant at the short incus process. Audiol Neurootol 2014;19:1–11. http://dx.doi.org/10.1159/000354981.

30. Huber AM, Veraguth D, Schmid S, et al. Tight stapes prosthesis fixation leads to better functional results in otosclerosis surgery. Otol Neurotol 2008;29:893–9. http://dx.doi.org/10.1097/MAO.0b013e318184f4f0.

31. Gan RZ, Wood MW, Dyer RK, et al. Mass loading on the ossicles and middle ear function. Ann Otol Rhinol Laryngol 2001;110(5 Pt 1):478–85.

32. Snik A, Cremers C. Audiometric evaluation of an attempt to optimize the fixation of the transducer of a middle-ear implant to the ossicular chain with bone cement. Clin Otolaryngol Allied Sci 2004;29:5–9.

33. Lenarz T, Weber BP, Issing PR, et al. Vibrant sound bridge system. A new kind hearing prosthesis for patients with sensorineural hearing loss. 2. Audiological results. Laryngorhinootologie 2001;80:370–80. http://dx.doi.org/10.1055/s-2001-15707.

34. Jenkins HA, Pergola N, Kasic J. Intraoperative ossicular loading with the Otologics fully implantable hearing device. Acta Otolaryngol 2007;127:360–4. http://dx.doi.org/10.1080/00016480601089424.

35. Gerard JM, Thill MP, Chantrain G, et al. Esteem 2 middle ear implant: our experience. Audiol Neurootol 2012;17:267–74. http://dx.doi.org/10.1159/000338689 ISSN: 1420-3030.

36. Zenner HP, Leysieffer H. Total implantation of the Implex TICA hearing amplifier implant for high-frequency sensorineural hearing loss: the Tübingen University experience. Otolaryngol Clin North Am 2001;34:417–46. http://dx.doi.org/10.1016/S0030-6665(05)70340-6.

37. Needham AJ, Jiang D, Bibas A, et al. The effects of mass loading the ossicles with a floating mass transducer on middle ear transfer function. Otol Neurotol 2005;26:218–24.

38. Cremers CW, Verhaegen VJ, Snik AF. The floating mass transducer of the Vibrant Soundbridge interposed between the stapes and tympanic membrane after incus necrosis. Otol Neurotol 2009;30:76–8. http://dx.doi.org/10.1097/MAO.0b013e31818f5790.

39. Hüttenbrink KB, Beutner D, Bornitz M, et al. Clip vibroplasty: experimental evaluation and first clinical results. Otol Neurotol 2011;32:650–3. http://dx.doi.org/10.1097/MAO.0b013e318218d180.

40. Shimizu Y, Puria S, Goode RL. The floating mass transducer on the round window versus attachment to an ossicular replacement prosthesis. Otol Neurotol 2010;32:98–103. http://dx.doi.org/10.1097/MAO.0b013e3181f7ad76.

41. Huber AM, Mlynski R, Müller J, et al. A new vibroplasty coupling technique as a treatment for conductive and mixed hearing losses: a report of 4 cases. Otol Neurotol 2012;33:613–7. http://dx.doi.org/10.1097/MAO.0b013e31824bae6e.

42. Zahnert T, Bornitz M, Hüttenbrink KB. Experiments on the coupling of an active middle ear implant to the stapes footplate. Adv Otorhinolaryngol 2010;69:32–7.

43. Kiefer J, Arnold W, Staudenmaier R. Round window stimulation with an implantable hearing aid (Soundbridge) combined with autogenous reconstruction of the auricle - a new approach. ORL J Otorhinolaryngol Relat Spec 2006;68:378–85. http://dx.doi.org/10.1159/000095282.

44. Osaki Y, Sasaki T, Kondoh K, et al. Implantation of a vibratory mass transducer on the round window: a report of two cases. Nippon Jibiinkoka Gakkai Kaiho 2008;111:668–71.

45. Baumgartner WD, Böheim K, Hagen R, et al. The vibrant Soundbridge for conductive and mixed hearing losses: European multicenter study results. Adv Otorhinolaryngol 2010;69:38–50. http://dx.doi.org/10.1159/000318521.

46. Beltrame AM, Martini A, Prosser S, et al. Coupling the vibrant Soundbridge to cochlea round window: auditory results in patients with mixed hearing loss. Otol Neurotol 2009;30:194–201.

47. Böheim K, Mlynski R, Lenarz T, et al. Round window vibroplasty: long-term results. Acta Otolaryngol 2012;132:1042–8. http://dx.doi.org/10.3109/00016489.2012.684701.

48. Streitberger C, Perotti M, Beltrame MA, et al. Vibrant Soundbridge for hearing restoration after chronic ear surgery. Rev Laryngol Otol Rhinol (Bord) 2009;130:83–8.

49. Gunduz B, Atas A, Bayazit YA, et al. Functional outcomes of Vibrant Soundbridge applied on the middle ear windows in comparison with conventional hearing aids. Acta Otolaryngol 2012;132:1306–10. http://dx.doi.org/10.3109/00016489.2012.702353.

50. Tringali S, Koka K, Deveze A, et al. Round window membrane implantation with an active middle ear implant: a study of the effects on the performance of round window exposure and transducer tip diameter in human cadaveric temporal bones. Audiol Neurootol 2010;15:291–302. http://dx.doi.org/10.1159/000283006.

51. Pau HW, Just T. Third window vibroplasty: an alternative in surgical treatment of tympanosclerotic obliteration of the oval and round window niche. Otol Neurotol 2010;31:225–7. http://dx.doi.org/10.1097/MAO.0b013e3181cc07fd.

52. Devèze A, Koka K, Tringali S, et al. Active middle ear implant application in case of stapes fixation: a temporal bone study. Otol Neurotol 2010;31:1027–34. http://dx.doi.org/10.1097/MAO.0b013e3181edb6d1.

53. Bellucci RJ, Fisher EG, Rhodin J. Ultrastructure of the round window membrane. Laryngoscope 1972;82:1021–6. http://dx.doi.org/10.1288/00005537-197206000-00010.

54. Su WY, Marion MS, Hinojosa R, et al. Anatomical measurements of the cochlear aqueduct, round window membrane, round window niche, and facial recess. Laryngoscope 1982;92:483–6.

55. Nakajima HH, Merchant SN, Rosowski JJ. Performance considerations of prosthetic actuators for round-window stimulation. Hear Res 2010;263:114–9. http://dx.doi.org/10.1016/j.heares.2009.11.009.

56. Arnold A, Kompis M, Candreia C, et al. The floating mass transducer at the round window: direct transmission or bone conduction? Hear Res 2010;263:120–7. http://dx.doi.org/10.1016/j.heares.2009.12.019.

57. Nakajima HH, Dong W, Olson ES, et al. Evaluation of round window stimulation using the floating mass transducer by intracochlear sound pressure measurements in human temporal bones. Otol Neurotol 2010;31:506–11. http://dx.doi.org/10.1097/MAO.0b013e3181c0ea9f.

58. Schraven SP, Hirt B, Gummer AW, et al. Controlled round-window stimulation in human temporal bones yielding reproducible and functionally relevant stapedial responses. Hear Res 2011;282:272–82. http://dx.doi.org/10.1016/j.heares.2011.07.001.

59. Ishii T, Takayama M, Takahashi Y. Mechanical properties of human round window, basilar and Reissner's membranes. Acta Otolaryngol Suppl 1995;519:78–82.

60. Arnold A, Stieger C, Candreia C, et al. Factors improving the vibration transfer of the floating mass transducer at the round window. Otol Neurotol 2010;31:122–8. http://dx.doi.org/10.1097/MAO.0b013e3181c34ee0.

61. Rajan GP, Lampacher P, Ambett R, et al. Impact of floating mass transducer coupling and positioning in round window vibroplasty. Otol Neurotol 2011;32:271–7. http://dx.doi.org/10.1097/MAO.0b013e318206fda1.

62. Rosowski JJ, Merchant SN. Mechanical and acoustic analysis of middle ear reconstruction. Am J Otol 1995;16:486–97.

63. Häusler R, Stieger C, Bernhard H, et al. A novel implantable hearing system with direct acoustic cochlear stimulation. Audiol Neurootol 2008;13:247–56. http://dx.doi.org/10.1159/000115434.

64. Bernhard H, Stieger C, Perriard Y. Design of a semi-implantable hearing device for direct acoustic cochlear stimulation. IEEE Trans Biomed Eng 2011;58:420–8. http://dx.doi.org/10.1109/TBME.2010.2087756.

65. Chatzimichalis M, Sim JH, Huber AM. Assessment of a direct acoustic cochlear stimulator. Audiol Neurootol 2012;17:299–308. http://dx.doi.org/10.1159/000339214.

66. Lenarz T, Zwartenkot JW, Stieger C, et al. Multicenter study with a direct acoustic cochlear implant. Otol Neurotol 2013;34:1215–25. http://dx.doi.org/10.1097/MAO.0b013e318298aa76.

67. Dumon T. Vibrant Soundbridge middle ear implant in otosclerosis: technique - indication. Adv Otorhinolaryngol 2007;65:320–2. http://dx.doi.org/10.1159/000098852.

68. Venail F, Lavieille JP, Meller R, et al. New perspectives for middle ear implants: first results in otosclerosis with mixed hearing loss. Laryngoscope 2007;117:552–5. http://dx.doi.org/10.1097/MLG.0b013e31802dfc59.

69. Kontorinis G, Lenarz T, Mojallal H, et al. Power stapes: an alternative method for treating hearing loss in osteogenesis imperfecta? Otol Neurotol 2011;32:589–95. http://dx.doi.org/10.1097/MAO.0b013e318213b0f1.

70. Schwab B, Salcher RB, Maier H, et al. Oval window membrane vibroplasty for direct acoustic cochlear stimulation: treating severe mixed hearing loss in challenging middle ears. Otol Neurotol 2012;33:804–9. http://dx.doi.org/10.1097/MAO.0b013e3182595471.

71. Beleites T, Neudert M, Beutner D, et al. Experience with vibroplasty couplers at the stapes head and footplate. Otol Neurotol 2011;32:1468–72. http://dx.doi.org/10.1097/MAO.0b013e3182380621.

72. Klein K, Nardelli A, Stafinski T. A systematic review of the safety and effectiveness of fully implantable middle ear hearing devices: the carina and esteem systems. Otol Neurotol 2012;33:916–21. http://dx.doi.org/10.1097/MAO.0b013e31825f230d.

73. Barbara M, Manni V, Monini S. Totally implantable middle ear device for rehabilitation of sensorineural hearing loss: preliminary experience with the Esteem, Envoy. Acta Otolaryngol 2009;129:429–32. http://dx.doi.org/10.1080/00016480802593505.

74. Maier H, Salcher R, Schwab B, et al. The effect of static force on round window stimulation with the direct acoustic cochlea stimulator. Hear Res 2013;301:115–24. http://dx.doi.org/10.1016/j.heares.2012.12.010.

75. Komori M, Yanagihara N, Hinohira Y, et al. Re-implantation of the Rion E-type semi-implantable hearing aid: status of long-term use and hearing outcomes in eight patients. Auris Nasus Larynx 2012;39:572–6. http://dx.doi.org/10.1016/j.anl.2011.12.003 cited By (since 1996) 0. ISSN: 03858146.

76. Yanagihara N, Suzuki J, Gyo K, et al. Development of an implantable hearing aid using a piezoelectric vibrator of bimorph design: state of the art. Otolaryngol Head Neck Surg 1984;92:706–12.

77. Zenner HP, Rodriguez Jorge J. Totally implantable active middle ear implants: ten years' experience at the University of Tübingen. Adv Otorhinolaryngol 2010;69:72–84. http://dx.doi.org/10.1159/000318524.

78. Abbass H, Kane M. Mechanical, acoustic and electromagnetic evaluation of the semi-implantable middle ear hearing device (SIMEHD). Ear Nose Throat J 1997;76:321–7.

79. Goll E, Dalhoff E, Gummer AW, et al. Concept and evaluation of an endaurally insertable middle-ear implant. Med Eng Phys 2013;35:532–6. http://dx.doi.org/10.1016/j.medengphy.2012.08.005.

80. Hough JV, Matthews P, Wood MW, et al. Middle ear electromagnetic semi-implantable hearing device: results of the phase II SOUNDTEC direct system clinical trial. Otol Neurotol 2002;23(6):895–903 ISSN: 1531-7129.

81. Silverstein H, Atkins J, Thompson JH Jr, et al. Experience with the SOUNDTEC implantable hearing aid. Otol Neurotol 2005;26:211–7 ISSN: 1531-7129.

82. Maniglia AJ, Ko WH. Semi-implantable middle ear electromagnetic hearing device for sensorineural hearing loss. Ear Nose Throat J 1997;76:333–8, 340–1.

83. Fay JP, Perkins R, Levy S, et al. Preliminary evaluation of a light-based contact hearing device for the hearing impaired. Otol Neurotol 2013;34:912–21. http://dx.doi.org/10.1097/MAO.0b013e31827de4b1.

84. Perkins R, Fay JP, Rucker P, et al. The EarLens system: new sound transduction methods. Hear Res 2010;263:104–13. http://dx.doi.org/10.1016/j.heares.2010.01.012.

Historical Development of Active Middle Ear Implants

Matthew L. Carlson, MD[a], Stanley Pelosi, MD[b], David S. Haynes, MD[c],*

KEYWORDS

- Middle ear implant(s) • Hearing rehabilitation • Sensorineural hearing loss
- Implantable hearing aids

KEY POINTS

- Over the last 20 years, there have been significant advances in active middle ear implant (AMEI) design.
- Many modern devices provide comparable objective audiometric performance with optimally fitted conventional hearing aids and afford a more natural, clear sound, with minimal feedback.
- Despite continued progress, the field of AMEIs is very young; there are still many theoretic benefits that have yet to be fully realized.
- With continued device innovation, expanding indications, and improvements in reimbursement, AMEIs will undoubtedly continue to develop.

INTRODUCTION

Hearing loss is one of the most common chronic disabilities and affects up to 48 million people in the United States.[1] Approximately 1 in 4 adults older than the age of 60 years suffer from bilateral hearing loss, most of which is not surgically reversible. Despite a high prevalence of hearing impairment, only 15% of hearing aid candidates use conventional aids on a regular basis, making hearing loss the single largest chronic sensory impairment that remains untreated.[2,3] This statistic seems surprising, because binaural hearing loss has been shown to significantly affect patient quality of life, leading to social isolation, anxiety, depression, and even cognitive decline.[4–6]

Financial and material support: no funding or other support was required for this study.
Conflict of interest to declare: the authors report no conflicts of interest concerning the information presented in this paper.
[a] Department of Otolaryngology-Head and Neck Surgery, Mayo Clinic, 200 First Street SW, Rochester, MN 55905, USA; [b] Department of Otolaryngology-Head and Neck Surgery, Thomas Jefferson University, Philadelphia, PA, USA; [c] Department of Otolaryngology-Head and Neck Surgery, The Bill Wilkerson Center for Otolaryngology & Communication Sciences, 7209 Medical Center East, South Tower, 1215 21st Avenue South, Nashville, TN 37232-8605
* Corresponding author.
E-mail address: david.haynes@vanderbilt.edu

Otolaryngol Clin N Am 47 (2014) 893–914
http://dx.doi.org/10.1016/j.otc.2014.08.004
0030-6665/14/$ – see front matter © 2014 Elsevier Inc. All rights reserved.

oto.theclinics.com

Common objections to hearing aid use frequently include cost of purchase and maintenance, social stigma associated with hearing aid use and concern over self-image, lack of audiometric benefit in those with severe loss or poor word recognition, and discomfort.[3,7,8]

The primary impetus for AMEI development is the desire to overcome many of the shortcomings that are inherent in conventional hearing aid design. To receive sufficient usable gain, patients with advanced hearing loss require a tight-fitting ear mold, which can lead to occlusion effect, discomfort, and ear canal irritation. Despite sophisticated sound processing strategies, distortion and feedback still plague even the best hearing aid designs at high output levels. AMEIs receive acoustic signal and directly stimulate the cochlea through coupling of the long process of the incus, stapes suprastructure, footplate, or round window. Because many AMEIs bypass the external ear canal and do not use a speaker for signal amplification, they effectively circumvent symptoms of occlusion effect and offer the potential for improved sound clarity and enhanced functional gain.

HISTORICAL GROUNDWORK FOR ACTIVE MIDDLE EAR IMPLANT DEVELOPMENT

Although there are significant variations in modern AMEI designs, all devices have substantial component overlap with conventional hearing aids, the primary differences being that a coupled mechanical transducer replaces the receiver, and at least 1 component is surgically implanted. Therefore, AMEI development has benefited significantly from improvements in hearing aid design, including ear mold integration, device ergonomics, component miniaturization, microchip technologies, advancements in speech processing, microphone technology, and battery design. Although a comprehensive review of conventional hearing aid history is outside the scope of this article, the most important advance to affect AMEI development began with the application of integrated circuit technology developed by Jack Kilby of Texas Instruments in 1958. Subsequent improvements such as the microprocessor, borrowed from the computer industry, permitted implementation of developing complex sound processing strategies. The first hearing aids with digital speech processing became commercially available in the 1980s. Most hearing aid users own a fully digital aid that is capable of flexible gain processing, multi-channel wide dynamic range compression, feedback suppression, and digital noise reduction.[9]

THE EARLY HISTORY OF ACTIVE MIDDLE EAR IMPLANT TECHNOLOGY

All modern electronic devices designed for hearing rehabilitation include several basic components: a microphone, power source, signal processor, and a specialized end component designed to deliver conditioned signal to a portion of the auditory system. Examples of a specialized end component include a cochlear implant electrode array, an auditory brainstem implant electrode pad, the acoustic receiver of air conduction hearing aids, and an osseointegrated screw for implantable bone conduction hearing aids. The primary component that distinguishes an AMEI from other designs is the transducer, containing an input sensor and output actuator, converting electrical signal into mechanical vibration. Although many types of mechanical transducers exist, devices used in middle ear surgery must be lightweight, energy efficient, reliable and durable, biocompatible, and operate with high fidelity. Over the last century, piezoelectric and electromagnetic-based transducers have emerged as suitable options for use in AMEI devices. The development of these technologies is discussed later.

Development of Electromagnetic-Based Middle Ear Transducers (Also Known as Electrodynamic)

Alvar Wilska,[10] a Finnish physiologist, is credited with the first attempt at mechanical stimulation of the auditory system through the use of an electromagnetic driver. In 1935, Wilska published the results of early experiments, in which he placed 10-mg iron pellets on the tympanic membrane and subjected them to a magnetic field generated by an electromagnetic coil inside an earphone. By adjusting the rate of oscillation, Wilska was able to reliably control the frequency of sound produced. He determined that vibratory amplitudes as small as ~ 0.1 nM (the diameter of a hydrogen ion) could elicit sound thresholds at 1000 Hz. Wilska himself participated in many of these early experiments, despite the discomfort that was generated from the heat and physical contact of the metal substrates on the tympanic membrane.

Subsequently, in 1959, Rutschmann[11] devised a method of fixing a tiny permanent magnet to the tympanic membrane at the umbo with water-soluble glue. By introducing an alternating current ranging between 0.1 and 3.0 A, pure tones between 2000 and 10,000 Hz could be generated. In his experiments, 2 individuals reported the ability to decipher an audio broadcast. Rutschmann realized early on that this technology carried a significant advantage over air conduction hearing aids for patients with advanced hearing loss by eliminating the problem of feedback at high output levels. In addition, he envisioned that with further refinement, this technology could bypass eroded ossicles or a diseased tympanic membrane and directly stimulate the inner ear through coupling of the oval or round window.

In the 1970s and 1980s, several researchers performed similar experiments with placement of a fixed magnet on the tympanic membrane outside the middle ear space. In 1973, Goode and Glattke[12] performed a series of experiments on 5 individuals using an Alnico V magnet fixed at the umbo, which was driven by an electromagnetic coil located on the postauricular skin. One of the 5 individuals was evaluated during a middle ear operation for tympanic neurectomy, allowing the investigators to examine differences in audition with magnet placement at the umbo, long process of the incus, and the oval window. From their work, the investigators found that tympanic membrane loading did not seem to significantly affect air conduction thresholds, and word recognition score performance using electromagnetic induction was comparable with conventional audiometric testing.

In 1988, Heide and colleagues[13] reported an important modification to previous studies by replacing a postauricular transducer with an in-the-canal electromagnetic induction coil located millimeters from a magnet fixed at the umbo. A mean functional gain of 17.5 dB was achieved, with no significant differences in word recognition compared with the users' own hearing aids. Similar to previous experiments, patients cited benefits including a more natural sound without feedback and improved performance in the presence of background noise.

Two types of electromagnetic-based systems have been developed: the electromagnetic and the noncontact electromagnetic configuration.[14] The noncontact electromagnetic design consists of a rare earth magnet, neodymium-iron-boron (NdFeB) or samarium-cobalt (SmCo), which is fixed to the tympanic membrane, ossicular chain, or round window membrane. A separate energizing coil, located millimeters away, creates a fluctuating magnetic field, which causes the magnet to vibrate in synchrony with incoming electrical signal, resulting in displacement of cochlear fluid and auditory stimulation. This configuration carries several theoretic advantages, including limited ossicular loading from the single small magnet, a unidirectional push of transmitted energy that replicates the natural action of middle ear energy transmission, and a noncontact coupling of the transducer. The primary disadvantage of this system is the short distance and coaxial alignment that must be kept between the transducer and the target magnet, because the strength of the magnetic field is lost inversely to the cube of the distance.

In contrast, the (contact) electromagnetic configuration incorporates an energizing coil and magnet together in a single housing, which is physically coupled to the ossicular chain or round window membrane. The fluctuating magnetic field results in magnet oscillation, creating vibrations. Although this design is usually more complex than the contactless electromagnetic system, it is generally more efficient and is not limited by the requirements of coaxial alignment and close proximity.

Development of Piezoelectric-Based Middle Ear Transducers

Piezoelectricity was first discovered by Jacques and Pierre Curie in 1880,[15] after observing that certain solid substrates developed an electrical charge proportional to an applied mechanical stress. The piezoelectric effect is a reversible event, whereby an applied electrical current can also result in a reproducible temporary deformity. In 1954, the metallic oxide-based piezoelectric material, lead zirconate titanate (PZT), was developed by Jaffe[16] and remains one of the most commonly used piezoelectric materials. When a voltage is applied, PZT crystals are deformed by approximately 0.1% of their original dimension. Thus, small PZT ceramics can be used as middle ear transducers to create predictable microvibrations to drive the ossicular chain.

Most piezoelectric transducers use a ceramic monomorph or a bimorph system. The monomorph design uses a single ceramic platform, which results in expansion and contraction after voltage application.[14] In contrast, the bimorph configuration uses 2 stacked crystals oriented in reverse polarities. When an electrical charge is applied, the platform bends, or oscillates, back and forth. In 1984, the RION Device was the first commercially approved piezoelectric-based AMEI to be implanted. Since this time, several additional AMEIs have used this technology, including the Implex TICA and the Envoy Esteem.

ELECTROMAGNETIC-BASED ACTIVE MIDDLE EAR IMPLANT SYSTEMS
Experimental Noncommercially Approved Device Designs

Semi-implantable middle ear electromagnetic hearing device
In 1986, Maniglia and colleagues[17] at Case Western Reserve University began investigating one of the first contactless electromagnetic-based AMEI systems. Through industry collaboration with Wilson Greatbatch (Clarence, NY), several successive models were developed and tested in animals. An early electromagnetic prototype incorporated placement of a target magnet on the stapes but required incudostapedial joint disarticulation. Realizing the drawbacks of permanently altering the ossicular chain in an otherwise healthy middle ear, the primary objective for subsequent designs was to develop an implant that did not require contact coupling, but rather, worked through a contactless system. Theoretically, such a design would allow the patient unimpeded use of a conventional hearing aid should the device fail, even without device explantation. Furthermore, because the actuator would not be rigidly connected to the ossicular chain, there would be less risk of ossicular erosion.

Early on, Maniglia and his coinvestigators determined that an electromagnetic system using an air-core actuator would provide the best functional characteristics to achieve their goal. Because of the significant technical obstacles associated with fully implantable designs, a semi-implantable device was created, using an external microphone, radiofrequency amplifier, transmitting antenna, and battery.[17] The external unit was designed to sit in a postauricular soft-tissue sling that was created using local rotational skin flaps. The internal component was to be implanted via mastoidectomy with atticotomy. A supporting frame was then secured to the mastoid cortex, and the transducer was placed within 0.5 to 1.0 mm of an NdFeB magnet, which was secured to the body of the incus with titanium-bone cement (Fig. 1).

Using a cat model, Maniglia and colleagues[17,18] found that the semi-implantable middle ear electromagnetic hearing device system did not interfere with normal acoustic hearing and afforded a mean 22 dB gain. Aside from antenna breakage, which was believed to be a problem unique to implantation within a cat, the device proved durable (9.6 months) and biocompatible. The results of these experiments led to US Food and Drug Administration (FDA) investigational device exemption approval for a limited clinical trial in May, 1996 for patients with moderate to severe sensorineural hearing loss (SNHL); however, to our knowledge, no further data were published regarding this device.

Round window electromagnetic system

Similar to several other contemporary AMEI investigators, Spindel and colleagues[19] recognized early on the importance of creating a coupling system that would bypass a healthy ossicular chain. Spindel's research team at the University of Virginia sought to develop a system that would provide direct cochlear activation through vibromechanical stimulation of the round window membrane. To investigate their prototype design, an animal study was devised, including 19 guinea pigs. Using a skin surface electromagnetic coil and an NdFeB target magnet on the round window membrane, the investigators reported a high degree of correlation between acoustic and electromagnetic stimulation using auditory brainstem response latency and amplitude data. Furthermore, the magnet did not seem to have any deleterious effects on normal acoustic hearing, and, because the design was not coupled to the ossicular chain, there was less risk of reverse energy transfer to the tympanic membrane, minimizing the possibility of reverse feedback. The investigators acknowledged difficulty with

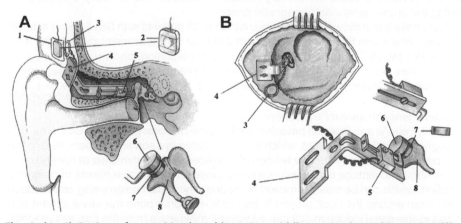

Fig. 1. (A, B) Design of a semi-implantable active middle ear implant: skin pocket (1), external processor (2), receiving antenna (3), supporting frame secured to mastoid cortex (4), implanted electronics package (5), electromagnetic transducer (6), magnet (7) attached to body of incus (8). (From Maniglia AJ, Ko WH, Rosenbaum M, et al. Contactless semi-implantable electromagnetic middle ear device for the treatment of sensorineural hearing loss. Short-term and long-term animal experiments. Otolaryngol Clin North Am 1995;28:128. Fig. 4A, B; with permission.)

determining the best method for permanent attachment of the magnet to the round window membrane. Although this prototype design has yet to be adapted to clinical applications, the investigators showed the feasibility of round window membrane coupling.

Electromagnetic ossicular augmentation device

In 1986, Kartush and Tos,[20] at the Michigan Ear Institute, collaborated with Smith & Nephew Richards, (Memphis, TN) to create an electromagnetic-based partially implantable AMEI that used an in-the-canal electromagnetic coil with a custom ear mold housing. These investigators participated in an FDA clinical trial using 3 different target magnetic configurations. In the first phase, 6 patients with bilateral sloping, high-frequency SNHL had a 30-mg to 45-mg SmCo magnet secured to the tympanic membrane with glue, approximately 2.5 to 3 mm from the ear canal transducer.[21] The results of this trial showed audiologic outcomes on par with optimally fitted hearing aids, and most patients reported no feedback, a more natural sound, and a subjective performance improvement when in environments with competing background noise.

In the second phase, an electromagnetic ossicular replacement device was created, using a total ossicular reconstruction prosthesis (TORP) design fitted with a target magnet. Patients were required to have mixed hearing loss associated with inactive chronic ear disease. In total, 7 national and 3 international coinvestigators participated. In their 1995 report, a preliminary summary of the first 50 implanted patients was published.[21] At the time of analysis, 26 patients were still using their device, 8 ears had device extrusion, 4 ossicular replacement devices were displaced, and 1 patient noted intermittent electromagnetic interference. Once again, audiologic outcomes were not significantly different from optimally fitted hearing aids; however, patients cited no problems with feedback, which permitted enhanced usable gain in addition to improved performance in noise. In a 2002 report, the long-term results of a 9-patient Danish cohort were published.[22] Although initial audiologic outcomes were promising, at last evaluation, none of the patients was using their device. In addition to device extrusion, the primary reason for nonuse was difficulty with properly fitting the in-the-canal electromagnetic driver.

The phase 3 trial allowed for the implantation of 10 patients with SNHL using a target magnet, which was fitted to the undersurface of the tympanic membrane. At the time of the last report,[20] 3 patients had undergone implantation, and no audiologic outcomes were provided. Although more than 50 patients were implanted using these technologies, device fitting remained problematic, and with time, funding was lost.

EarLens tympanic contact transducer

In 1993, Perkins and Shennib patented the EarLens platform (Redwood City, CA). This design used an SmCo magnet, which was embedded in a soft silicone lens held to the tympanic membrane by surface tension after placement of a thin layer of mineral oil.[23] The primary advantage of this technology includes a less invasive means of magnetic fixation, which can be easily removed if needed. The initial design using an induction loop worn around the neck proved to be inefficient, prompting the development of a small in-the-canal induction coil placed several millimeters from the EarLens magnet. In 1996, a feasibility study was performed,[24] including 7 patients evaluated over a 3-month period. Tympanic membrane loading resulted in a ~5 dB loss; however, the maximum mean functional gain was 25 dB. There was no evidence of tympanic membrane irritation over the course of follow-up. A 16-patient follow-up study was published in 2010, using a refined in-the-canal electromagnetic coil and a 9-mg gold-coated disk magnet.[23] Again, the EarLens system was well tolerated, and the ear canal transducer provided patients with enough output to reach thresholds of 60 dB HL. A recent modification includes use of a behind-the-ear processor containing a low-power laser diode that emits coded infrared light, which, in turn, activates a small tympanic membrane electrokinetic actuator embedded in the soft lens platform.[25] At the time of writing, the EarLens system has not sought FDA clearance.

MED-EL Vibrant Soundbridge (formerly the Symphonix device)
The Vibrant Soundbridge (VSB) was the first FDA approved AMEI system for implantation of patients with SNHL, receiving approval in August, 2000.[2] Initial device development began in 1996 and was pioneered by Geoffrey Ball, a cofounder of Symphonix Devices (San Jose, CA). The relatively slow adoption of the VSB after FDA approval led to the dissolution of Symphonix, and in March, 2003, the VSB technology was purchased by MED-EL (Innsbruck, Austria). Several years later, the VSB received the European Union CE Marking for treatment of conductive and mixed hearing loss in adults (2008) and children (2009).

The VSB consists of 2 primary components: an external audio processor and a surgically implanted vibrating ossicular prosthesis (VORP).[2] The external audio processor contains a microphone, signal processor, telemetry coil, and a replaceable battery, all housed within in a single unit. The external unit is designed to sit against the postauricular skin, in the hairline, through magnetic attraction with the implanted receiver. The original external device, the Vibrant P, used analogue processing. Since that time, several generations of digital processors have been developed; the current fifth-generation design, the Amadé Audio Processor, offers a directional microphone, 3 programs to choose from, and several new sound processing features designed to minimize wind noise and attenuate background noise. The device uses a nonrechargeable zinc air battery, which requires replacement approximately once per week.

The implanted VORP comprises 3 functional units, including a receiver, demodulator unit, and an electromechanical floating mass transducer (FMT); the footprint of the implanted system is similar to modern cochlear implants (**Fig. 2**). The implanted receiver, containing a magnet and coil, collects signal data transcutaneously, which are processed in a demodulator unit and are subsequently sent through a flexible conductor link to the transducer. The 2.3 × 1.6 mm FMT consists of 2 polymide-coated gold coil wires wrapped around a hermetically sealed titanium casing. Within the transducer housing sits an SmCo magnet, which is suspended by a set of silicone elastomer springs. The application of an alternating current induces a magnetic field that stimulates movement of the encased magnet, resulting in vibration of the entire FMT unit. The VORP can be implanted via a mastoidectomy with facial recess approach or through transmeatal access.[26] With either approach, a postauricular incision is performed to create a well and trough for the implanted receiver and demodulator. Most commonly, the FMT is attached to the incus with a prosthesis clip; however, several other FMT coupling options exist, including round window, oval window, and TORP or partial ossicular reconstruction prosthesis vibroplasty.

Since its clinical debut, there have been more than 50 publications on the VSB, making it the most heavily clinically studied AMEI. Most data show good short-term and long-term audiometric performance comparable with optimally fit hearing aids; however, subjective patient-centered outcome data consistently favor the VSB over conventional hearing aids.[27]

Ototronix Maxum (formerly the SOUNDTEC direct system)
In the early 1980s, the Hough Ear Institute, located in Oklahoma City, began a series of experiments that led to the development of the SOUNDTEC Direct Drive Hearing

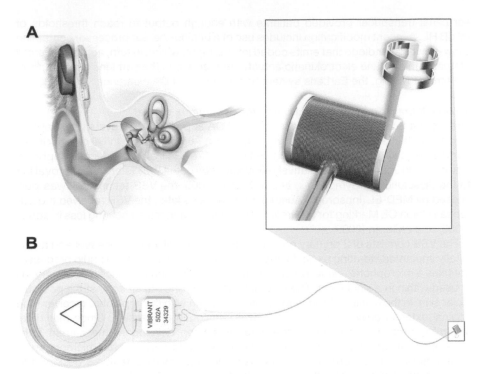

Fig. 2. (A) The Vibrant Soundbridge middle ear implant system. (B) Implanted VORP containing an FMT. (*Courtesy of* MED-EL, Durham, NC; with permission.)

System, becoming only the second AMEI to receive FDA approval, in September, 2001.[28] Initial research focused on the development of an optimal target magnet design. Various NdFeB magnets were tested in several locations, including a donut-shaped design over the stapes suprastructure, a magnet placed between the malleus handle and promontory, and one positioned between the stapes capitulum and the malleus. In 1988, 5 patients with moderate SNHL were implanted with a target magnet placed at the incudostapedial joint.[29] Oxidation of the magnet occurred as a result of moisture exposure during preimplant preparation. A redesigned implant using an SmCo rare earth magnet was reimplanted in 4 of the 5 original patients. However, despite audiologic benefit, 6-month testing showed a significant decline in unaided high-frequency hearing thresholds; therefore, device explantation was required.[30]

Over the following 6 years, improvements in device design led to an FDA-sanctioned phase 1 clinical trial in 1998, including 5 patients with moderate to moderately severe SNHL.[31] Upgrades from the earlier prototypes included a stronger and lighter magnet, a hermetically sound titanium laser welded canister, and a wire clip for attachment at the incudostapedial joint, designed to provide optimal coaxial alignment with the in-the-canal electromagnetic coil. Implantation involves a ~45-minute procedure, using a transcanal approach. The incudostapedial joint is carefully divided, and gentle back-traction on the incus is performed while the ring wire is slipped over the capitulum. The incus is then repositioned over the stapes capitulum to allow for fibrous union. Patients are usually fitted with an ear mold coil assembly with a behind-the-ear processor 10 weeks after surgery (Fig. 3). The results of the first clinical trial showed a 50% (~15 dB) improvement in functional gain, and ~20% improvement in speech recognition scores over the patients' previously worn hearing

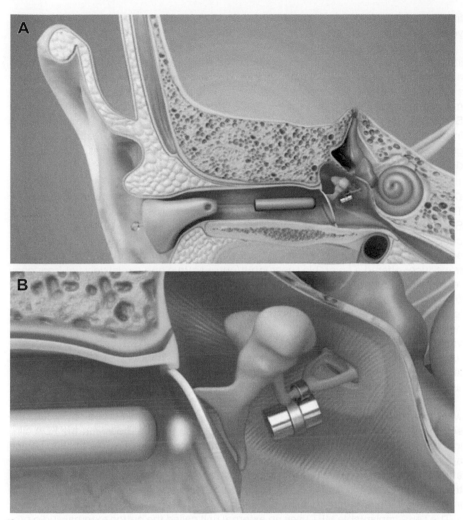

Fig. 3. (*A, B*). Semi-implantable Maxum Hearing Implant using an open-fit, completely-in-the-canal electromagnetic sound processor. (*Courtesy of* Ototronix, Spring, TX; with permission.)

aids.[31] Furthermore, subjective measures, including sound quality and patient satisfaction, were superior to conventional amplification.

This initial success led to a multicenter phase 2 clinical trial, the results of which were published in 2002.[32] A total of 103 patients were implanted at 10 sites within the United States. The basic elements of the phase 1 trial device were preserved; however, the target magnet was replaced with a lighter 27-mg NdFeB magnet to improve on threshold losses resulting from ossicular loading, seen in the phase 1 trial. Compared with optimally fit hearing aid performance, implanted patients received a mean 7.9-dB improvement in functional gain and a 5.3% increase in speech discrimination. Similarly, subjective measures evaluating sound quality, presence of occlusion and feedback, and device preference favored the SOUNDTEC device. Because there was only a 4-dB shift in hearing thresholds after implantation, presumably from incudostapedial joint separation and ossicular loading, patients could use a conventional aid if preferred.

Despite the initial success of the SOUNDTEC device, with more than 600 patients implanted, the device was voluntarily removed from the market in 2004 to investigate a problem of an audible rattle that patients were experiencing while the sound processor was not in place. This problem was believed to result from movement of the target magnet at its single point of fixation. In 2009 Ototronix, LLC (Spring, TX) purchased the SOUNDTEC technology, and the device was re-released as the Maxum Hearing Implant after incorporating several notable upgrades, including a miniaturized integrated digital processor and coil and a self-crimping Nitinol wire that obviates incudostapedial joint separation.

Otologics semi-implantable middle ear transducer and fully implantable Carina

The development of the partially implantable Middle Ear Transducer (MET) Ossicular Stimulator and the fully implantable Carina system began in the 1970s with research conducted by Fredrickson and colleagues[33] at Washington University in St Louis, Missouri. Early preclinical experiments[34] showed that their prototype electromagnetic transducer offered a favorable linear input/output curve and a relatively flat frequency response. Testing was subsequently performed on 11 rhesus monkeys using auditory brainstem response and distortion product otoacoustic emission data. Short-term and long-term results showed that the vibromechanical stimulation from the electromagnetic transducer was comparable with natural acoustic hearing; furthermore, it provided high fidelity of frequency transfer and had little effect on normal acoustic function after implantation. An early feasibility study using the MET Ossicular Stimulator was performed on 5 patients, confirming good sound quality and improved audiometric performance.

In 1996, the MET technology was sold to Otologics (Boulder, CO), shortly after which phase 1 clinical trials began in the United States and Europe. By 2000, the semi-implantable MET was commercially available in Europe; however, the FDA clinical trials were never completed. Recognizing the large costs associated with device approval in the United States, Otologics sought to concentrate monetary and research efforts toward the ongoing development of the Carina, a fully implantable version of the MET. In 2006, the Carina received the European Union CE Mark for implantation in patients with moderate to severe SNHL.

The semi-implantable MET uses an external unit called the button external audio processor, containing a microphone, battery, signal processor, and transmitter.[34] The implanted portion consisted of a receiver, electronics package, and electromagnetic driver. The MET transducer is implanted through a limited transmastoid atticotomy centered over the posterosuperior ear canal to gain access to the incus and malleus. Next, a mounting system is fixed to the skull with screws, and a 1-mm-deep hole is made in the body of the incus using a laser. The MET Ossicular Stimulator transducer system is introduced; the receiving coil and electronics package is placed in a recessed well, and the aluminum oxide tip of the transducer probe is inserted into the receiving hole in the incus (**Fig. 4**). The fully implantable Carina uses the same electromagnetic transduction system, but includes an implantable battery, sound processor, and receiving coil for device charging and programming.[35] A separate microphone that is connected to the implanted sound processor is placed in a postauricular subcutaneous pocket.

In 2004, Jenkins and colleagues[36] published the results of a large multicenter study, including 282 patients who were implanted with the semi-implantable MET in Europe and the United States. There were no significant air conduction or bone conduction threshold shifts after implantation, showing minimal effect from ossicular loading

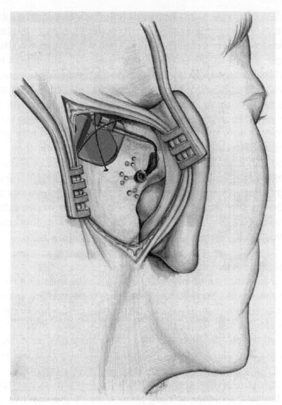

Fig. 4. Surgical implantation of the semi-implantable MET. (From Kasic JF, Fredrickson JM. The Otologics MET ossicular stimulator. Otolaryngol Clin North Am 2001;34:512. Fig. 8; with permission.)

and no evidence of inner ear trauma. Functional gain and speech recognition scores were similar to best-fit hearing aids. Subsequently, in 2008, Jenkins and colleagues[35] published the 1-year results of a phase 1 clinical trial investigating the fully implantable Carina system in 20 patients. After implantation, there were no significant differences in bone conduction thresholds; however, air conduction thresholds were slightly worse at 2-month, 3-month, and 6-month evaluations. Pure tone averages and monaural word recognition scores favored the patients' walk-in-aided condition, whereas subjective patient perceived benefit was better for the implant-aided condition. By 12 months, several notable complications occurred, including partial device extrusion in 3 ears, loss of external communication in 2, and increased charging times in 7 patients; together 8 of 20 devices were explanted. Ongoing clinical investigations in the United States were discontinued, and the company filed chapter 11 bankruptcy in July, 2012; the technology was subsequently purchased by Cochlear (Sydney, Australia) in September of the same year.

PIEZOELECTRIC-BASED ACTIVE MIDDLE EAR IMPLANT SYSTEMS
Experimental Noncommercially Approved Device Designs

Dresden University of Technology implantable hydroacoustic transducer
In 2001, Hüttenbrink and colleagues[37,38] published the results of an implantable hydroacoustic transducer prototype tested in human cadaveric temporal bone

specimens using laser Doppler vibrometry. Noting that normal physiologic amplitudes of tympanic membrane movement range from molecule-sized vibrations with routine sound transmission to 1 mm with ambient air pressure changes, and that the undistributed ossicular chain is built to absorb large fluctuations through joint movement, Hüttenbrink theorized that many AMEI designs carried a fundamental flaw in the ossicular coupling mechanism. That is, a coupler that is rigidly fixed to the actuator may induce remodeling of the contact point, causing reduced effectiveness over time. The newly proposed design includes a 10-mm hollow piezoceramic cylinder transducer, with 1 end connected to the sound processing unit and the other free end containing a thin latex membrane behaving as a balloon tip. The system is then filled with water, and the soft balloon tip is placed in contact with the ossicles or round window membrane. Hüttenbrink and colleagues reported that the novel design not only transmitted mechanical energy effectively but could also successfully receive vibratory signal from the ossicles, showing the added potential to act as an implantable microphone. Although a notable contribution to AMEIs, to our knowledge, this device has not yet been tested in vivo.

Semicircular canal piezoelectric vibrator

One of the primary limitations of early AMEI designs was the need to disarticulate the ossicular chain to couple the transducer. This issue is particularly germane to patients with pure SNHL, because existing hearing loss would be compounded by conductive deficit should the device fail. Recognizing this drawback, several investigators pursued methods to stimulate the inner ear and not disturb an intact middle ear hearing mechanism. One such system was pioneered by Welling and Barnes[39] at the Ohio State University.

Before the description of the stapedectomy procedure for otosclerosis by John Shea Jr in 1956, lateral canal fenestration procedures were used to create a second functioning mobile window in the labyrinth, bypassing a fixed stapes footplate. Inspired by earlier reports, Welling and Barnes devised a piezoelectric biomorph that could activate the auditory system via vibromechanical stimulation of a semicircular canal fenestration (**Fig. 5**). The investigators first performed the procedure on 4 cats and subsequently on a patient who was undergoing a posterior semicircular canal occlusion under light sedation for intractable benign paroxysmal positional vertigo. In their experiments, the investigators showed the feasibility of this approach. Despite piezoelectric stimulation of the posterior canal, the human patient denied vertigo, and no nystagmus was elicited. To our knowledge, no further applications of the technology have been reported.

University of Bordeaux implantable piezoelectric transducer

Similar to Welling and Parnes, Dumon and colleagues,[40] at the University of Bordeaux, France, sought to design a system that would sidestep the need to irreversibly damage an intact functioning ossicular chain. Short-term and long-term feasibility experiments were performed using an implantable system consisting of a piezoelectric biomorph with a short rod and platinum ball placed against the round window of guinea pigs. Cochlear stimulation was assessed using auditory evoked potentials and direct eighth nerve action potential monitoring. These investigators determined that round window coupling was both feasible and safe. Specifically, round window vibrostimulation resulted in stable and reproducible responses with input-to-output curves comparable with acoustic stimulation. Histologic studies showed no evidence of injury to the round window membrane or middle ear. These early animal experiments determined that although oval window stimulation was

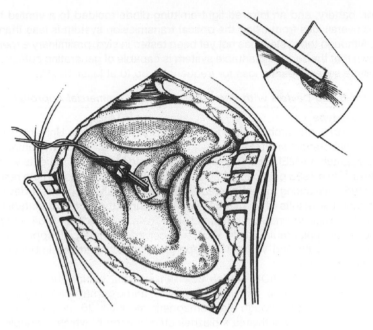

Fig. 5. Stimulation of the posterior semicircular canal using a piezoelectric transducer after canal fenestration. (*From* Welling DB, Barnes DE. Acoustic stimulation of the semicircular canals. Otolaryngol Clin North Am 1995;28:212. Fig. 4; with permission.)

possible, incudostapedial joint coupling was more efficient, prompting a redesign for human cadaveric temporal bone studies.

A human prototype was developed and tested in 12 temporal bones. After a standard intact canal wall mastoidectomy and large facial recess, a pliable bayonet-shaped adjustable fixing strut was secured to the skull. The free end included a thin plate-shaped extension, which was designed to slip between a disarticulated incudostapedial joint. Because of the slender design of the vibrating plate, the incus does not require subluxation or removal, so that if the device requires explantation, the ossicular chain can be easily mended. Testing showed promising results; however, the investigators noted that the size of the device may preclude placement in patients with contracted mastoid cavities. Since Dumon and colleagues'[40] 1995 publication, no reports have been published regarding application of this technology to living individuals.

Piezoelectric round window implant with infrared optical signal
In 2011, the University of Tübingen began developing a piezoelectric-based AMEI that used a microactuator, located on the round window, which could receive power and signal transmission through an infrared optical transmitter located in the ear canal.[41] This design is notable because it is the first piezoelectric-based AMEI that can be implanted endaurally without mastoidectomy. The system is made possible by a small 1.7-mm prototype PZT actuator connected to a photodiode array. Because of the size restrictions imposed from placement within the round window niche and the energy requirements needed to generate sufficient vibrational amplitudes, a unimorph slotted-disk actuator was developed, containing a passive silicone layer stacked over an active piezoelectric platform. The external unit contains a microphone, sound

processor, battery, and an infrared light-emitting diode molded to a vented tip. The estimated overall loss from using the optical transmission system is less than 25 dB at 1 kHz. Although the system has not yet been tested in vivo, preliminary experiments have shown that the semi-implantable system is capable of generating sufficient force to rehabilitate severe hearing loss for frequencies up to at least 10 kHz.

Piezoelectric-Based Devices with Current or Previous Commercial Approval

RION Device E-type

Beginning in 1978, researchers from Ehime University and Teikyo University in Japan worked in collaboration with RION (Tokyo, Japan) to develop a fully implantable and a partially implantable AMEI using a piezoelectric-based system for patients with mixed hearing loss.[42] In a 1983 publication, Suzuki and colleagues[43] reported the results of a 6-month study evaluating in vivo characteristics of a totally implantable device in 15 cats. Although the results of this study were promising, the semi-implantable design was the only device to undergo human clinical trials beginning in 1984. In October, 1993, the semi-implantable RION Device received commercial approval by the Department of Health and Welfare of Japan, supporting partial reimbursement by health insurance carriers.[44]

The semi-implantable RION Device uses an external behind-the-ear processor, which houses a microphone, amplifier, processor, and external coil.[45] Signal is transmitted transcutaneously through electromagnetic induction to the internal receiving coil, which subsequently activates a piezoelectric biomorph, which is coupled to the stapes (**Fig. 6**). Implantation can be performed in an intact canal wall or a canal wall down cavity; thus, patients with existing open mastoid cavities can still undergo implantation but require ear canal closure. Whether performed in a canal wall up or canal wall down cavity, the basic elements of surgery are similar. A mastoidectomy is performed to permit room for implantation of the internal device and to gain access to the middle ear space. A stabilizing plate, connected to the piezoelectric biomorph, is fixed with titanium screws to the cortex of the squamosal temporal bone. The free end of the piezoelectric transducer is placed in light contact with the stapes capitulum and is attached using a small hydroxyapatite tube. If the stapes suprastructure is missing, a prosthesis can be adapted and interposed between the transducer and footplate.

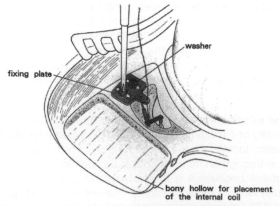

Fig. 6. Surgical implantation of the partially implantable RION Device using an intact canal wall technique. (*From* Yanagihara N, Gyo K, Hinohira Y. Partially implantable hearing aid using piezoelectric ceramic ossicular vibrator. Results of the implant operation and assessment of the hearing afforded by the device. Otolaryngol Clin North Am 1995;28:92. Fig. 5; with permission.)

The first generation of the partially implantable RION Device E-type was implanted in 28 patients with mixed hearing loss between 1984 and 1989, and all but 1 subject experienced significant hearing improvement with device use.[42] Long-term, 17 total patients experienced complications: 8 developed severe eustachian tube dysfunction, tympanic membrane retraction pockets, or early cholesteatomas; 3 patients underwent device removal after transducer exposure; 4 patients required device explantation because of postauricular mastoid-cutaneous fistulas, which were attributed to the thickness of the internal coil; and 4 subjects lost benefit from their device because of progressive SNHL or from disruption of the interposed hydroxy-apatite tube.

A second version of the RION Device was developed in response to the complications seen with the first design.[42] Improvements included a thinner internal coil, a more robust lead wire, and a more powerful external unit, affording an average 10-dB improvement in gain. In addition, modifications of the intact canal wall procedure were made to decrease the risk of tympanic membrane retraction, including lateralization of the tympanic membrane and cartilage reinforcement. A total of 11 patients were implanted with the second-generation device, beginning in 1990; 1 developed a retroauricular fistula and 2 required revision surgery for cholesteatoma. In both groups, a hearing level improvement of 30 dB was achieved immediately after surgery, and none of the patients experienced SNHL that was attributable to implantation or device use. Most patients reported high satisfaction from reduced feedback and more natural, clear sound compared with their conventional hearing aids. In 2005, the RION Device was discontinued, because the company was unable to maintain a sufficient profit in Japan's socialized medical insurance system.[46]

Implex totally implantable cochlear amplifier

The totally implantable cochlear amplifier (TICA) was conceived by Leysieffer and Zenner at the University of Tübingen in 1988 and was developed in cooperation with Implex AG Hearing Technology (Munich, Germany) between 1993 and 1997.[47,48] Although no longer available, the TICA LZ3001 is noteworthy as the first available fully implantable AMEI, receiving the CE Marking for use in Europe in 1998. The motivation to design a fully implantable system was to allow users total freedom and complete concealment. Patients can swim, participate in sports, and even sleep while their device remains on. In addition, because the TICA uses a subcutaneous sound sensor near the tympanic membrane, it takes full advantage of natural sound filtering from the pinna and ear canal.

The fully implantable design of the TICA made optimal component design especially critical; the TICA required a compact size, durable hermeticity, efficient energy use, options for battery charging, optimal microphone placement and design, and reliable componentry; because the device is totally implanted, any modifications beyond processor programming necessitate revision surgery. The TICA LZ3001 consists of 3 implantable modules: the processor containing the battery and digitally programmable audio processor, the membrane receptor acting as the microphone, and a piezo-electric transducer.[48] During early development, it was determined that a circular heteromorph piezoelectric actuator would provide the most energy-efficient method of vibrostimulation. This design is different from the rod-shaped biomorph used by the RION Device. The TICA uses a hermetically sealed titanium casting that provides a nonferrous, lightweight, durable biocompatible housing. The sound processor uses an integrated rechargeable battery, which can be reenergized through use of the induction coil. The TICA provides a battery life of approximately 50 hours, requiring roughly 2 hours for a full charge. With average use, the battery requires replacement every 3 to 5 years.

Implantation is performed through a postauricular canal wall up mastoidectomy. Trephination of the posterior canal wall, close to the tympanic membrane, is performed so that the microphone sensor can be placed directly underneath the ear canal skin to receive acoustic signal.[48] Next, a fixing plate designed to stabilize the actuator is screwed to the skull, and a titanium coupling rod, an extension of the transducer, is linked to the ossicular chain (**Fig. 7**). The TICA was designed with 3 coupling options: the long process of the incus using a clip, the body of the incus using a conical indentation and ionomeric cement, or the footplate using a conventional piston prosthesis attached to the coupling rod.

One problem that arose in several patients was noise feedback. While the device was activated, ossicular vibrations could be transmitted to the tympanic membrane, leading to sound in the ear canal that was picked up by the subcutaneous ear canal sound sensor. To remove the potential for reverse feedback, a portion of the neck of the malleus could be resected, thereby decoupling the tympanic membrane and distal ossicular chain.[48] In addition, because the entire device was placed in the postauricular/mastoid space, the device was too large for patients with small contracted mastoids, preventing implantation in an estimated 14% of ears.[47] For this reason, it was recommended that patients undergo preoperative computed tomography to assess mastoid pneumatization.

The results of a phase 3 clinical trial were published in 2004, including 20 patients with bilateral moderate to severe SNHL.[49] At 6 months after implantation, 3 patients did not receive benefit, whereas the remaining 17 showed improved word recognition scores, functional gain, and sound localization over the preoperative unaided condition. Despite receiving commercial approval in Europe, the device lost financial support from Implex AG Hearing Technology. After bankruptcy, the technology was purchased by Cochlear, with the intent of adapting the fully implantable technology to future cochlear implant designs.

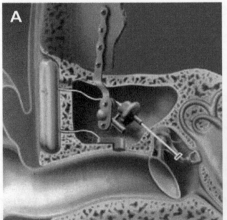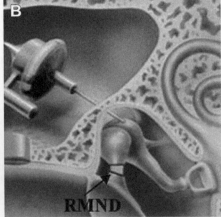

Fig. 7. (*A, B*) Surgical implantation of the TICA with transducer coupling to the body of the incus and reversible malleus neck dissection (RMND). (*From* Zenner HP, Leysieffer H. Total implantation of the Implex TICA hearing amplifier implant for high-frequency sensorineural hearing loss: the Tubingen University experience. Otolaryngol Clin North Am 2001;34:430. Fig. 14A, B; with permission.)

Envoy Esteem

In 1995, St Croix Medical, now Envoy Medical Corporation (St Paul, MN), was founded, with the goal of designing a fully implantable device that did not use a microphone or speaker. Initial development focused on creating a dual piezoelectric biomorph transducer system, including a sensor placed on the proximal ossicular chain and an actuator positioned on the stapes.[50,51] Javel and colleagues[52] published the results of early in vivo experiments examining a variety of piezoelectric transducers implanted in cats. The performance of transducers positioned at the umbo was assessed using laser Doppler vibrometry, and auditory brainstem responses, cochlear microphonics, and compound action potentials were used to compare threshold sensitivity, signal quality, frequency response, and output levels of a transducer located on the stapes capitulum. This study showed that a sensor transducer placed on the umbo could create an effective bandwidth output of greater than 8 kHz and that cochlear potentials created by an appropriately designed piezoelectric transducer were similar to acoustically elicited responses.

The Esteem II system is composed of a hermetically sealed titanium dual sound processor with an integrated nonrechargeable lithium battery, along with 2 separate piezoelectric transducers.[50,53] The device is placed through a postauricular transmastoid approach with extended facial recess. The sound processor is implanted in a 2-mm bony well and stabilized with suture, similar to how a cochlear implant receiver-stimulator package is secured. The distal 3 mm of the long process of the incus is removed with a laser to prevent feedback, because the receiver and stimulator are both located along the ossicular chain. Both transducers are then fixed in the mastoid cavity with hydroxyapatite cement and the sensor interface is linked to the body of the incus using glass-ionomer cement, and the driver is cemented to the capitulum of the stapes (**Fig. 8**). The nonrechargeable battery has an estimated 5-year to 9-year life span and requires a small surgical procedure for replacement after expiration. An external device controls volume and programming.

The results of a 7-patient phase 1 clinical trial were published in 2004.[51] After implantation, there were 4 patients who failed to gain benefit, resulting from a breach in hermeticity at either the sensor or driver. After revision surgery, there were 5 patients who could participate in audiometric performance testing 2 months after surgery. In these patients, functional gain and speech reception testing were similar to conventional air conduction hearing aids; word recognition scores were better than preoperative unaided scores but did not improve over optimally fitted hearing aids.

Two phase 2 trials were subsequently performed between 2004 and 2009; the results of the second phase 2 trial, including 57 patients from 3 centers, was reported by Kraus

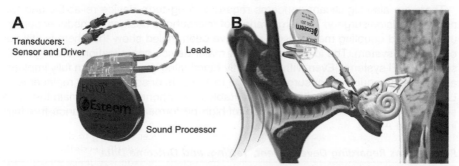

A
Transducers: Sensor and Driver
Leads
Sound Processor

B

Fig. 8. (*A, B*) The fully implantable Envoy Esteem system using a piezoelectric sensor and actuator. (*Courtesy of* Envoy Medical, St Paul, MN; with permission.)

and colleagues[53] in 2011. Audiometric performance at 12 months after surgery, comparing the best-fit aided condition and the implant-aided condition, showed an Speech recognition threshold (SRT) improvement of ~12 dB, pure tone average gain of 27 dB, and word recognition score improvement of ~22%; no changes in bone conduction were noted. Furthermore, quality of life data showed that most implantees believed that their device was equal or better than their previous conventional aid, using questionnaires assessing self-confidence, lifestyle, clarity of sound, and speech understanding in noise. Three patients experienced a delayed facial palsy that subsequently resolved, and 3 patients required revision surgery because of limited benefit. After phase 2 clinical trials within the United States, the FDA granted device approval in March, 2010. Concurrent clinical investigations in Europe led to CE Marking in 2006.

ONGOING CHALLENGES FACING ACTIVE MIDDLE EAR IMPLANT DEVELOPMENT
Anticipated Versus Realized Benefits

The initial motivation for the development of AMEIs was to provide an alternative to conventional hearing aids for patients with moderate to severe hearing loss. Although most commercially approved devices show a satisfactory risk profile, several series have reported a high rate of implant extrusion, temporary and permanent facial paralysis, and device malfunction. To justify the greater cost and increased risk associated with AMEIs, there must be a substantial benefit to the user compared with conventional air conduction hearing aids. The theoretic advantages of an implantable hearing aid include improved functional gain, reduced risk of feedback, enhanced sound quality, greater speech understanding in noise, improved concealment, lack of occlusion, and greater freedom to lead an active lifestyle. Although, clearly, substantial improvements have been made over the past several decades, many of these theoretic advantages have not yet been realized. For example, most contemporary studies fail to show a statistically significant improvement in functional gain and word recognition scores over optimally fit hearing aids.[27] Realizing the significant challenges of creating a fully implantable AMEI, most companies have focused on developing partially implanted models. Because these devices contain an external microphone, sound processor, and battery, they do not carry significant advantages over conventional hearing aids with regard to concealment or freedom. Furthermore, many semi-implantable devices use an in-the-canal component, which may still create occlusion effect and canal irritation. The few devices that use a fully implantable design frequently require partial ossicular resection to minimize reverse feedback. After device failure, these patients may be left with a considerable conductive hearing loss, which compounds preexisting hearing loss.

There are also significant concerns regarding long-term device reliability and the need for revision surgery. The large variety of microphone designs, transducer configurations, and coupling mechanisms that have been trialed show that there is still not one perfect system. The long-term risks of major device complications are high with several AMEI systems. Even with a perfectly functioning device, modern fully implantable systems require minor surgery every 5 to 10 years or so for battery replacement. Limitations in battery capacity and implantable microphone designs remain the most significant obstacles to the development of high-performance, maintenance-free fully implantable AMEIs.

Reservations Regarding Development, Testing, and Outcome Data

Concerns have been raised by the medical community that much monetary support for clinical investigations has been secured through private investors, which may create unconscious bias in clinical study design and data analysis. Because AMEIs are marketed as an alternative to conventional hearing aids, future clinical studies must compare these technologies with preoperative performance using an optimally fitted hearing aid. Furthermore, the use of independent investigators, without potential competing interests, may help minimize the risk of study bias. Many studies contain significant methodological weaknesses that make it difficult to decipher the true benefit of device implantation.

Financial Challenges

Beyond the major challenges associated with device design, AMEI companies face significant financial obstacles. First, the current market niche for AMEIs is limited, and there is still little awareness among many audiologists and general otolaryngologists regarding the indications and benefits of implantation. Most devices target patients with moderate to moderately severe SNHL. AMEIs are not recommended for patients with mild hearing impairment. In addition, implantation of patients with severe SNHL is problematic, because many experience progressive losses, which may exceed the output capabilities of their implanted device. As hearing aid technologies continue to improve and audiometric candidacy criteria for cochlear implantation progressively relax, competition within the AMEI market will increase. Several AMEI companies have received approval for implantation in patients with conductive and mixed hearing loss, thereby increasing the number of eligible patients.

One of the most substantial challenges facing AMEI companies is the significant upfront expense of research and development for commercial device approval. To recuperate costs, the average price of an AMEI with surgery ranges from approximately $9000 to $30,000, whereas the cost for a high-end pair of conventional hearing aids is approximately $6000. Insurance reimbursement remains inconsistent, and the cost of implantation is too high for many private payers.

SUMMARY

Over the last 20 years, there have been significant advances in AMEI design. Many modern devices provide comparable objective audiometric performance with optimally fitted conventional hearing aids and afford a more natural, clear sound, with minimal feedback. Despite continued progress, the field of AMEIs is very young; there are still many theoretic benefits that have yet to be fully realized. With continued device innovation, expanding indications, and improvements in reimbursement, AMEIs will undoubtedly continue to develop.

REFERENCES

1. Lin FR, Niparko JK, Ferrucci L. Hearing loss prevalence in the United States. Arch Intern Med 2011;171:1851–2.
2. Ball GR. The Vibrant Soundbridge: design and development. Adv Otorhinolaryngol 2010;69:1–13.
3. Kochkin S, MarkeTrak V. "Why my hearing aids are in the drawer": the consumers' perspective. Hear J 2000;53:34–42.
4. Lin FR, Metter EJ, O'Brien RJ, et al. Hearing loss and incident dementia. Arch Neurol 2011;68:214–20.
5. Mick P, Kawachi I, Lin FR. The association between hearing loss and social isolation in older adults. Otolaryngol Head Neck Surg 2014;150(3):378–84.
6. Mener DJ, Betz J, Genther DJ, et al. Hearing loss and depression in older adults. J Am Geriatr Soc 2013;61:1627–9.

7. Haynes DS, Young JA, Wanna GB, et al. Middle ear implantable hearing devices: an overview. Trends Amplif 2009;13:206–14.
8. Mills M. Hearing aids and the history of electronics miniaturization. IEEE Ann Hist Comput 2011;33:24–45.
9. Kim HH, Barrs DM. Hearing aids: a review of what's new. Otolaryngol Head Neck Surg 2006;134:1043–50.
10. Wilska A. Eine Methode zur Bestimmung der Hörschwellenamplituden des Trommelfells bei verschiedenen Frequenzen. Skandinavisches Archiv für Physiologie 1935;72:161–5 [in German].
11. Rutschmann J. Magnetic audition auditory stimulation by means of alternating magnetic fields acting on a permanent magnet fixed to the eardrum. IRE Trans Med Electron 1959;6:22–3.
12. Goode RL, Glattke TJ. Audition via electromagnetic induction. Arch Otolaryngol 1973;98:23–6.
13. Heide H, Tatge G, Sander T, et al. Development of a semi-implantable hearing device. In: Suzuki I, Hoke M, editors. Middle Ear Implant: Implantable Hearing Aids. Basel: Karger; 1988. p. 32–43.
14. Ko WH, Zhu WL, Kane M, et al. Engineering principles applied to implantable otologic devices. Otolaryngol Clin North Am 2001;34:299–314.
15. Diamantis A, Magiorkinis E, Papadimitriou A, et al. The contribution of Maria Sklodowska-Curie and Pierre Curie to nuclear and medical physics. A hundred and ten years after the discovery of radium. Hell J Nucl Med 2008;11:33–8.
16. Fujishima S. The history of ceramic filters. IEEE Trans Ultrason Ferroelectr Freq Control 2000;47:1–7.
17. Maniglia AJ, Ko WH, Rosenbaum M, et al. Contactless semi-implantable electromagnetic middle ear device for the treatment of sensorineural hearing loss. Short-term and long-term animal experiments. Otolaryngol Clin North Am 1995;28:121–40.
18. Maniglia AJ, Ko WH, Garverick SL, et al. Semi-implantable middle ear electromagnetic hearing device for sensorineural hearing loss. Ear Nose Throat J 1997;76:333–8, 340–1.
19. Spindel JH, Lambert PR, Ruth RA. The round window electromagnetic implantable hearing aid approach. Otolaryngol Clin North Am 1995;28:189–205.
20. Kartush JM, Tos M. Electromagnetic ossicular augmentation device. Otolaryngol Clin North Am 1995;28:155–72.
21. McGee TM, Kartush JM, Heide JC, et al. Electromagnetic semi-implantable hearing device: phase I. Clinical trials. Laryngoscope 1991;101:355–60.
22. Caye-Thomasen P, Jensen JH, Bonding P, et al. Long-term results and experience with the first-generation semi-implantable electromagnetic hearing aid with ossicular replacement device for mixed hearing loss. Otol Neurotol 2002;23:904–11.
23. Perkins R, Fay JP, Rucker P, et al. The EarLens system: new sound transduction methods. Hear Res 2010;263:104–13.
24. Perkins R. Earlens tympanic contact transducer: a new method of sound transduction to the human ear. Otolaryngol Head Neck Surg 1996;114:720–8.
25. Fay JP, Perkins R, Levy SC, et al. Preliminary evaluation of a light-based contact hearing device for the hearing impaired. Otol Neurotol 2013;34: 912–21.
26. Vibrant Soundbridge the implantable hearing system: information for surgeons for incus and round window vibroplasty. MED-EL GmbH; 2007. Available at: http://www.medel.com/data/pdf/28031.pdf. Accessed January 12, 2014.

27. Kahue CN, Carlson ML, Daugherty JA, et al. Middle ear implants for rehabilitation of sensorineural hearing loss: a systematic review of FDA approved devices. Otol Neurotol 2014;35(7):1228–37.
28. Hough J, Vernon J, Johnson B, et al. Experiences with implantable hearing devices and a presentation of a new device. Ann Otol Rhinol Laryngol 1986;95:60–5.
29. Hough J, Dormer KJ, Baker RS, et al. Middle ear implantable hearing device: ongoing animal and human evaluation. Ann Otol Rhinol Laryngol 1988;97:650–8.
30. Baker RS, Wood MW, Hough JV. The implantable hearing device for sensorineural hearing impairment. The Hough Ear Institute experience. Otolaryngol Clin North Am 1995;28:147–53.
31. Hough JV, Dyer RK Jr, Matthews P, et al. Semi-implantable electromagnetic middle ear hearing device for moderate to severe sensorineural hearing loss. Otolaryngol Clin North Am 2001;34:401–16.
32. Hough JV, Matthews P, Wood MW, et al. Middle ear electromagnetic semi-implantable hearing device: results of the phase II SOUNDTEC direct system clinical trial. Otol Neurotol 2002;23:895–903.
33. Fredrickson JM, Coticchia JM, Khosla S. Ongoing investigations into an implantable electromagnetic hearing aid for moderate to severe sensorineural hearing loss. Otolaryngol Clin North Am 1995;28:107–20.
34. Kasic JF, Fredrickson JM. The Otologics MET ossicular stimulator. Otolaryngol Clin North Am 2001;34:501–13.
35. Jenkins HA, Atkins JS, Horlbeck D, et al. Otologics fully implantable hearing system: phase I trial 1-year results. Otol Neurotol 2008;29:534–41.
36. Jenkins HA, Niparko JK, Slattery WH, et al. Otologics middle ear transducer ossicular stimulator: performance results with varying degrees of sensorineural hearing loss. Acta Otolaryngol 2004;124:391–4.
37. Huttenbrink KB, Zahnert TH, Bornitz M, et al. Biomechanical aspects in implantable microphones and hearing aids and development of a concept with a hydroacoustical transmission. Acta Otolaryngol 2001;121:185–9.
38. Hüttenbrink K. Implantierbare Hörgeräte für hochgradige Shwerhörgkeit. HNO 1997;45:737–48 [in German].
39. Welling DB, Barnes DE. Acoustic stimulation of the semicircular canals. Otolaryngol Clin North Am 1995;28:207–19.
40. Dumon T, Zennaro O, Aran JM, et al. Piezoelectric middle ear implant preserving the ossicular chain. Otolaryngol Clin North Am 1995;28:173–87.
41. Goll E, Dalhoff E, Gummer AW, et al. Concept and evaluation of an endaurally insertable middle-ear implant. Med Eng Phys 2013;35:532–6.
42. Yanagihara N, Sato H, Hinohira Y, et al. Long-term results using a piezoelectric semi-implantable middle ear hearing device: the RION Device E-type. Otolaryngol Clin North Am 2001;34:389–400.
43. Suzuki J, Kodera K, Yanagihara N. Evaluation of middle-ear implant: a six-month observation in cats. Acta Otolaryngol 1983;95:646–50.
44. Suzuki J, Kodera K, Nagai K, et al. Partially implantable piezoelectric middle ear hearing device. Long-term results. Otolaryngol Clin North Am 1995;28:99–106.
45. Yanagihara N, Gyo K, Hinohira Y. Partially implantable hearing aid using piezoelectric ceramic ossicular vibrator. Results of the implant operation and assessment of the hearing afforded by the device. Otolaryngol Clin North Am 1995;28:85–97.
46. Komori M, Yanagihara N, Hinohira Y, et al. Re-implantation of the RION E-type semi-implantable hearing aid: status of long-term use and hearing outcomes in eight patients. Auris Nasus Larynx 2012;39:572–6.

47. Maassen MM, Lehner R, Leysieffer H, et al. Total implantation of the active hearing implant TICA for middle ear disease: a temporal bone study. Ann Otol Rhinol Laryngol 2001;110:912–6.
48. Zenner HP, Leysieffer H. Total implantation of the Implex TICA hearing amplifier implant for high frequency sensorineural hearing loss: the Tubingen University experience. Otolaryngol Clin North Am 2001;34:417–46.
49. Zenner HP, Limberger A, Baumann JW, et al. Phase III results with a totally implantable piezoelectric middle ear implant: speech audiometry, spatial hearing and psychosocial adjustment. Acta Otolaryngol 2004;124:155–64.
50. Kroll K, Grant L, Javel E. The envoy totally implantable hearing system, St Croix Medical. Trends Amplif 2002;6:73–80.
51. Chen DA, Backous DD, Arriaga MA, et al. Phase 1 clinical trial results of the envoy system: a totally implantable middle ear device for sensorineural hearing loss. Otolaryngol Head Neck Surg 2004;131:904–16.
52. Javel E, Grant IL, Kroll K. In vivo characterization of piezoelectric transducers for implantable hearing AIDS. Otol Neurotol 2003;24:784–95.
53. Kraus EM, Shohet JA, Catalano PJ. Envoy Esteem totally implantable hearing system: phase 2 trial, 1-year hearing results. Otolaryngol Head Neck Surg 2011;145:100–9.

Vibrant Soundbridge Rehabilitation of Conductive and Mixed Hearing Loss

Jan-Christoffer Lüers, MD, Karl-Bernd Hüttenbrink, MD*

KEYWORDS

- Vibrant soundbridge • Implantable hearing aid • Hearing implant • Middle ear
- Conductive hearing loss • Mixed hearing loss

KEY POINTS

- There is growing evidence for the effectiveness and safety of the VSB in patients with conductive and mixed hearing loss.
- The indications for implantation of a VSB are primarily related to intolerance of a CHA.
- A wide range of FMT coupling methods have been developed, which may result in similar acoustic outcomes.
- Complications are rare and mainly related to insufficient functional hearing gain with the need to reposition the FMT in the round window niche.
- Studies indicate that the VSB can provide functional hearing gains at least as good as those achieved with CHA.

INTRODUCTION

The Vibrant Soundbridge (VSB; Med-El, Innsbruck, Austria) is a partially implantable active middle ear transducer system. Since its introduction into clinical practice about 15 years ago it has become the world's most often used active middle ear implant.[1] The outer component of the VSB, comprised of a microphone, audio processor, battery, transmitter coil, and magnet, processes incoming acoustical signals to an amplitude-modulated signal and delivers these transcutaneously to the inner VSB component. The inner component, or vibrating ossicular prosthesis (VORP), is comprised of an antimagnet, receiver unit, conductor link, and the floating mass transducer (FMT). The inner component is manufactured with a left- and right-sided version. After the signal is received and demodulated, it is sent to the FMT via the

Department of Otorhinolaryngology, Head and Neck Surgery, University of Cologne, Kerpener Street 62, Building 23, Cologne 50924, Germany
* Corresponding author.
E-mail address: huettenbrink.k-b@uni-koeln.de

Otolaryngol Clin N Am 47 (2014) 915–926
http://dx.doi.org/10.1016/j.otc.2014.08.002
0030-6665/14/$ – see front matter © 2014 Elsevier Inc. All rights reserved.

conductor link. The FMT is the core technology and key component of the VSB. It consists of a titanium housing with a coil and a magnet in close physical proximity to one another. In a set of biasing elements, the magnet and housing vibrate relative to one another, thus causing vibrations in direct response to the externally generated electric signal. When the FMT is attached to a mobile structure (ossicles, inner ear window) these vibrations can be transferred and the target organ (cochlea) is stimulated.[2] Hence, instead of acoustic energy, the VSB delivers mechanical energy to the cochlea, stimulating the inner ear fluids.

The VSB was originally designed in the late 1990s solely for patients with sensorineural hearing loss.[3] For this purpose, the FMT is coupled to the incus' long process via a small titanium clip. Analyzing the audiometric results of the first clinical trial it was found that the VSB could "also be used to treat conductive hearing loss."[4] The versatile possibilities of the surgical placement of the device because of its single anchor point attachment to the middle ear helped to explore alternative coupling methods for the FMT (length of 2.3 mm, diameter of 1.6 mm, mass weight of 25 mg), and with these, the application of the VSB has expanded to patients with conductive and mixed hearing loss.[5]

CANDIDACY FOR SURGERY

The first implantation of a VSB for sensorineural hearing loss was performed in 1996. After alternative coupling methods were discovered, the VSB is now also used to rehabilitate patients with conductive and mixed hearing loss.[1]

Currently, there is no clear evidence that the VSB is superior to conventional hearing aids (CHA) in functional qualities, such as hearing gain or threshold improvement.[6] Furthermore, there is large variance in the functional gain obtained in different patients, suggesting high variability in the effectiveness of the FMT coupling.[7] Hence, the implantation of a VSB cannot be indicated solely from the audiometric results, and currently the indications are mainly of a medical or cosmetic nature. Thus, if a patient has an indication for a CHA, but the application of this is not possible because of medical reasons, such as chronic external otitis or intolerance of an ear mold, then the VSB is a recommendable option for hearing rehabilitation.

In most cases of conductive hearing loss, a VSB is implanted into patients with a history of chronic otitis media with or without cholesteatoma. Normally, the VSB is only considered after conventional tympanoplasty and ossiculoplasty with a partial or total middle ear prosthesis has failed (ie, if application of a conventional middle ear prosthesis has not led to a satisfactory hearing result).

Although not a decisive indication parameter, audiologic prerequisites do exist for VSB candidates. For patients with conductive or mixed hearing loss, the bone conduction should not be worse than 45 to 65 dB within the frequencies 500 to 4000 Hz as recommended by the Med-El company (**Fig. 1**). There is not a speech discrimination criterion for the implantation of a VSB, but functional hearing outcome depends on this parameter. Although patients with a poor preoperative discrimination score of less than 40% (unaided) may show improvement with the VSB, patients with a discrimination score of 50% to 70% and higher are likely better candidates and long-term performance is likely to be better.[8] If there is a near normal hearing threshold on the contralateral ear, then this may influence the acceptance of a VSB, because some of these patients will not report a high subjective benefit. Hence, the indication of a VSB for unilateral hearing loss should be discussed individually.

Whether or not a VSB should be implanted in children, is open for debate. Since 2009, the VSB has approval in Europe for patients younger than 18 years. Following

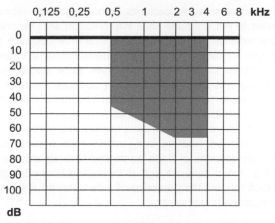

Fig. 1. Indication zone for VSB in patients with conductive or mixed hearing loss as recommended by the manufacturer; bone conduction should be within the shaded area. If the bone-conduction is better than 20dB, then the inherent ground noise of the VSB processor might be heard by a patient and hence, indication should be carefully discussed here.

a statement by an international consensus paper[9] the VSB has already been implanted in newborns.[10] Because the middle ear structures are fully developed at the time of birth and because the VSB uses a single-point attachment in the middle ear, patient growth is not expected to change the VSB performance over time. However, the limitations for a postimplant magnetic resonance imaging (MRI) scan are more restrictive in children, and it is recommended to carefully weigh the pros and cons of the VSB against all alternative therapies before implantation in children.[9] Preconditions for VSB implantation as recommended by the authors are listed in **Table 1**.

Table 1	
Preconditions for VSB implantation as recommended by the authors	
Preconditions for VSB Implantation	**Comment**
Suitable audiometric performance with bone conduction within the designated zone (see **Fig. 1**)	Indication zone is different for patients with sensorineural hearing loss
Stable inner ear function	Definition unclear
Either no benefit from CHA or no possibility to wear these	Severe malformations of the outer ear, recurrent external otitis and otorrhea, intolerance of the ear mold, and so forth
Exclusion of cholesteatoma; no signs of acute inflammation in the middle ear	Risk for labyrinthitis, risk for revision surgery, and so forth
Magnetic resonance imaging of the brain (optional)	Scan for cerebral pathologies before surgery because application of this imaging technique is limited after VSB implantation
High-resolution computed tomography of the temporal bone (optional)	Scan for cholesteatoma presence or signs of malformations
Acceptable language skills	Important for accommodation and tuning of audio processor
Realistic expectations of the hearing benefits	Final hearing result is not predictable
Psychological and emotional stability	

The VSB has been implanted in patients with congenital microtia or ear canal atresia.[11–14] It is wise to not combine VSB implantation with reconstructive surgery of the auricle or the external ear canal at the same time because the latter suffers from a significant rate of complications, which may harm the functionality of the VSB. However, for those patients suffering from pure conductive hearing loss, bone-anchored hearing aids are the first option because they are easier to apply, not putting the middle ear structures and inner ear function at risk during implantation and because they yield similar functional results.

At the authors' institution, children are initially offered a nonsurgical solution with a soft-band bone conduction hearing aid, which has proved its effectiveness. Currently, in adults, acceptance of bone-anchored hearing aids has improved after the introduction of a transcutaneous signal delivering (BoneBridge [Med-El, Innsbruck, Austria]), which renders the presence of a percutaneous fixture requiring daily cleaning and maintenance unnecessary.

PREOPERATIVE PLANNING AND PREPARATION

Some precautions must be considered before a VSB implantation. Patients being considered for implantation of an active hearing implant should have stable bone- and air-conduction thresholds. However, a generally accepted definition for "stable auditory thresholds" does not exist. A bone-conduction threshold not having deteriorated more than 15 dB in two consecutive frequencies within 12 months before implantation is suggested by the authors.[15]

Pure tone audiometry with appropriate masking and speech audiometry are highly recommended diagnostic tools before a VSB implantation. If the hearing performance cannot be determined with sufficient certainty by subjective audiometry, then objective audiometry (eg, auditory brainstem responses) is mandatory. Unlike the situation with passive middle ear prostheses for ossiculoplasty, tympanometry plays no key role for the VSB because its function is independent of the middle ear aeration. The testing of stapedial reflexes is reserved for specific cases, such as patients with otosclerosis where a VSB is implanted together with a stapes piston.[1,16]

Before a VSB implantation, a high-resolution computed tomography of the temporal bone is recommended to check the correct position of the anatomic structures of the inner ear, middle ear, and mastoid and to estimate the thickness of the parietal skull bone. Normally, VSB implantation is preceded by some sort of middle ear surgery with surgical exploration of the ear, and thus the intraoperative status of the ear is known to the surgeon. In these cases a new computed tomography scan is normally not necessary. Because most of the patients underwent several previous middle ear surgeries, earlier procedures must be respected and prior surgery reports should be collected and studied beforehand.[15]

Because an implanted VSB limits MRI of the brain, it might be advisable to scan for cerebral pathologies, if suspected, before VSB implantation. Although studies have shown that MRI examinations of up to 1.5 T likely do not present a serious risk of harm to the patient or damage to the VSB, a dislocation of the FMT is possible during MRI, and also image artifact will occur.[17]

A VSB should only be implanted in ears with no active inflammation and no cholesteatoma.[15] If cholesteatoma disease can be completely removed without concern of recurrence, then it is, in principle, possible to perform the eradication of the disease and the implantation of a VSB in one surgical session. However, a two-stage concept is probably used more often, where the initial cholesteatoma surgery with ossiculoplasty is done first. If this attempt fails because of insufficient hearing gain, and if

CHA are not desired or tolerated, then active middle ear implants become a reasonable option.

Further preparations are similar to other middle ear and temporal bone surgery (eg, routine blood examination). Naturally, the patient should be thoroughly informed about the device, its mode of operation, visual nature, and its potentials and limitations. Informed consent must be obtained from the patient before surgery where additional to common risks at middle ear surgery, the points of dependence of an external component, possible technical failure of the device, insufficient hearing gain, and MRI limitations should be discussed.

Regarding the required materials, it is advisable to have a backup implant available for the operation, which can be used if the first implant turns out to be defective or damaged during surgery. All commercially available titanium couplers for the VSB (clip or bell coupler for the stapes, TORP, or oval window [OW] coupler and round window [RW] coupler) should be on hand for the surgery, even if their use is not expected.

A VSB may be implanted bilaterally, but it is recommended to verify the acceptance and functional gain at one side (preferably the ear with the worse hearing) first and then have the other ear implanted in a separate second surgery.

SURGICAL TECHNIQUE
Procedural Approach

The procedural approach is similar to cochlear implant surgery and mainly consists of a mastoidectomy combined with a pathway to the middle ear cavity. Differences in the procedural approach depend on patient anatomy, disease, and surgeon preference. A retroauricular incision is needed to drill the implant bed in the parietal bone. The manufacturer provides silicone dummies that help to drill the exact size of the bed for the demodulator. A half-open bony channel can help to lock the demodulator in position. If the implant bed is drilled deep enough, then usually no additional stabilization with absorbable sutures is needed.[18] If necessary, the skin flap above the implant must be thinned out to ensure appropriate communication between the implant magnet and the audio processor magnet, postoperatively.

In most cases, the conductor link with the FMT runs through the mastoid, and hence a mastoidectomy is needed. If a VSB is placed in patients with a canal wall down mastoid cavity, it is recommended to partially obliterate the cavity first in a separate staged surgery. Partial or complete mastoid cavity obliteration helps protect the electrode from exposure and may help dry a chronically draining and mucosalized mastoid cavity.[19] Additionally, the electrode cable should be covered with thick cartilage plates to prevent electrode migration similar to cochlear implant surgery. Contingent on the success of this surgery to create a small and dry mastoid cavity, a VSB may be implanted at a second-stage surgery.

If the mastoid cavity is dry but large or shows deep retraction pockets, then a partial obliteration with bone pate is still highly recommended before VSB implantation because the risk for infection at the surgery site or the implant is believed to be greater with a large mastoid cavity.

If the chances for a dry external ear canal and functional middle ear are considered poor, and if there is a significant hearing impairment, then a total obliteration of the ear is recommended. This includes removal of the middle ear mucosa, tympanic membrane, and skin; plugging of the mastoid, middle ear, and eustachian tube with fat or local muscle flaps; and oversew of the ear canal. Here, the mastoid is again partly obliterated with bone pate, but the middle ear space is covered with cartilage to provide room for a later VSB placement (or cochlear implantation).

If the implantation is combined with repair of the tympanic membrane, then cartilage slices can be thicker than 0.5 mm, which is otherwise regarded as a good compromise between sufficient mechanical stability and low acoustic transfer loss in passive tympanoplasty.[20] Because the function of the VSB is independent of a vibrating tympanic membrane, cartilage slices of full thickness ($\sim$ 1 mm) can be used to achieve a stable coverage of the tympanic cavity.

In a canal wall up technique, the conductor link either runs through the mastoid antrum or through a posterior tympanotomy (facial recess) to the tympanic cavity. Particularly in cases of RW vibroplasty, it is recommended to provide a posterior tympanotomy with maximal lowering of the facial nerve spur to get a wide access to the RW niche. The removal of the RW's bony lip is an obligatory surgical step in RW vibroplasty. The drilling procedure can be hazardous and must be done with great caution to avoid any contact to the membrane with the risk of an irreversible acoustic trauma of the inner ear. If the RW is not sufficiently exposed, then the FMT contacts the RW's bony lip with the risk of a suboptimal coupling to the inner ear. Some surgeons use a cartilage chip or a piece of fascia to improve the contact between the FMT and RW membrane. Fascia, however, may be subject to shrinking, and thus the contact between FMT and RW may become loose in the long-term with decreasing hearing gain. These fundamental problems with RW vibroplasty are best addressed with the RW coupler, which centers the FMT and provides optimized contact of the FMT to the RW membrane (**Fig. 2**). The RW coupler helps to overcome the diameter mismatch of the FMT (1.6 mm), unprepared RW niche (1.3–1.6 mm), and RW membrane (0.8–1.75 mm).[21,22] Besides optimizing the contact between FMT and RW, the RW coupler minimizes surgical risks, because the bony lip of the RW must not be maximally drilled away (bony rim flush to the membrane). To stabilize the position of FMT and titanium coupler assembly to the membrane, cartilage chips in conjunction with fibrin glue are placed around and below the FMT, resulting in a cylindrical encasement of the assembly, which vibrates like a piston toward the membrane. Unlike the situation with passive middle ear prosthesis, fibrin glue can be used with any combination of FMT and coupler because the function of the FMT is independent of an aerated middle ear.

If the stapes is intact and mobile (without tympanosclerotic fixation) then a bell or clip vibroplasty is the treatment of choice. Compared with the bell coupler, the clip coupler seems to be a better alternative because of its more stable connection to the stapes head, and thus it offers better protection against dislocation[23] especially considering the additional weight of the FMT (25 mg) that is attached on top of the stapes and coupling device (**Fig. 3**).

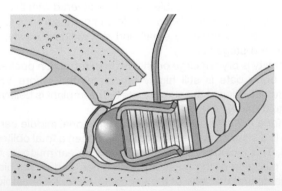

Fig. 2. The RW coupler optimizes the contact between FMT and round window membrane and reduces drilling procedures and thus the risk of damage to the inner ear.

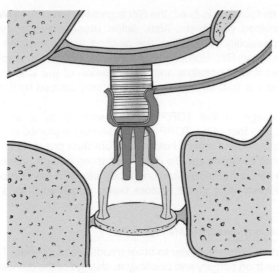

Fig. 3. The clip coupler requires a stable and mobile stapes. The FMT can have contact to the tympanic membrane, which is stabilized with a thick slice of cartilage. This provides for a direct sound transmission using the FMT as an active and passive prosthesis at the same time.

If the stapes suprastructure is missing, but the stapes footplate is stable and mobile, then an OW vibroplasty with a TORP coupler is the best option.[24] A prerequisite for this is a stable but mobile stapes footplate.[25] Similar to a passive TORP, an efficient transfer of vibrations correlates to an optimal and long-term stable placement of the columella-like OW coupler and here the use of a cartilage shoe for centralizing the prosthesis on the footplate has proved to be a reliable method (**Fig. 4**).[26]

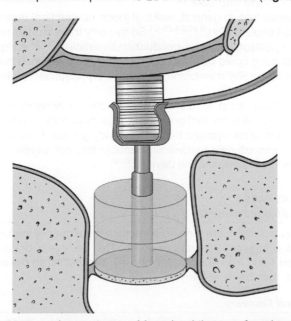

Fig. 4. The OW or TORP coupler requires a stable and mobile stapes footplate. It is best secured with a cartilage shoe. Like the clip coupler it can also serve as a passive prosthesis.

If the stapes or its footplate is fixed, the RW approach using the RW coupler comes into play as described previously. Also, failed otosclerosis or tympanosclerosis surgery with no possibility to improve the hearing with a revision stapes surgery may be treated with an RW vibroplasty, if CHA cannot be applied. Here, the OW should be reclosed first, if possible, with explantation of the stapes piston to avoid leakage of the inner ear fluid through the stapedotomy caused by the FMT vibrations on the RW.

Recently, the usage of the TORP coupler serving as a stapes piston was described.[27] Here, the foot of the TORP-FMT assembly is placed into a stapedotomy while a silicon ring between titanium holder and footplate prevents the assembly from deeper insertion into the inner ear. To date, only three patients have undergone this procedure, which needs further evaluation, especially with the combination of inner-ear opening in chronic otitis media, before being considered as a true alternative coupling method.

Potential Complications and Their Management

The VSB implantation risks are similar to other middle ear surgeries. Technical failures with the need for revision surgery and possibly exchange of the device are possibilities of which the patient must be informed about preoperatively. In general, intraoperative complications are rare in VSB implantation[8,16,28] but unfortunately the complication rate is not reported in all studies.[29] Surgical orientation in the mastoid can be difficult because of missing anatomic landmarks after numerous middle ear surgeries. Malformations, adhesions and scar tissue, and the presence of passive tympanoplasty assemblies with scar tissue formation bear higher risks for subluxation of the stapes or opening the inner ear with resultant deafness and vertigo. Previous disease or ear surgery might have resulted in an exposed and unprotected facial nerve. It is recommended to smooth down any sharp edges of the mastoid so that they do not harm the conductor link of the VSB later.[15]

Most studies show that, in general, residual (bone conduction) hearing remains unchanged after VSB implantation.[8,23,24,28–31] So far, only three studies reported considerable changes in postsurgical bone-conduction thresholds.[32–34] A significant decline of the bone conduction could be attributed to either noise-induced hearing loss or to physical damage to the RW membrane, both possibly sustained while drilling out the RW membrane.[1,33]

Minor complications, such as damage to the chorda tympani nerve, temporary facial nerve palsy, hematomas, vertigo, and tinnitus, similar to conventional "passive" tympanoplasty, have been reported by various study groups. Infection at the implant region should be immediately treated with antibiotics, but severe infections might eventually require explantation of the device.[29,33]

POSTPROCEDURAL CARE
Medical and Audiology Follow-Up

Routine follow-up includes pure tone audiometry with testing of the bone conduction and regular tuning fork and nystagmus tests. The ear canal dressing is normally removed between 1 and 3 weeks postoperatively, depending on the extent of ear canal and tympanic membrane surgery.

Rehabilitation and Recovery

The fitting of the audio processor takes place after wound healing has finished and when the postoperative edema of the skin has diminished. The audio processor's magnet is available in four different strengths depending on the patient's need in terms of thickness of skin and hair. The housing of the audio processor is available in four different colors and normally the patient decides on a color matching his or her hair. There are three variants with different output gain (high, low, standard) to reach the best benefit for the patient. Normally the fine tuning takes several visits to the audiologist with multiple audiometric tests to find the best settings for each patient. Depending on country-specific circumstances, the fitting process is arranged and executed by the clinic or at the local audiologist.

SURGICAL AND HEARING OUTCOMES

Real long-term studies with large sample sizes are not yet available for the VSB in conductive or mixed hearing loss. To date, the longest reported outcomes are at 15 months follow-up.[31] Most studies are of a retrospective, nonrandomized, and noncontrolled design; none of them reach a level of evidence better than 2b.[35] When describing audiometric results, many authors report the patients' "functional hearing gain" or just display the aided sound-field thresholds, which leaves open the question of how much energy is needed for this amplification and hence the maximum output levels. As a further difficulty, the term "functional hearing gain" is used nonuniformly, and it is not always clear whether the aided sound-field thresholds (or speech perception) were compared with the unaided situation preoperatively or postoperatively. Furthermore, possible confounders of the hearing result (duration of deafness, severity of hearing loss, type of pathology) are rarely addressed in the literature, and thus it is difficult to judge their impact.[29,35] As a result, because of the heterogeneity of studies, a current true comparison of VSB studies or even a meta-analysis is difficult, if not impossible.[29] Nevertheless, all studies on VSB in mixed or conductive hearing loss consistently report great improvements in terms of "functional gain" and speech recognition compared with the unaided situation, and hence the VSB can be considered a very effective treatment.[1,5,8,28–31,33,36]

Unfortunately, attempts to compare the hearing results of the VSB at conductive or mixed hearing loss with "best fitting" CHA in a convincing manner are rare.[1] A requirement for such studies is a prospective design with a detailed report of long-range systematic attempts for optimal fitting of CHA (with testing of multiple different types and brands). Additionally, the amplification and signal-to-noise ratios for CHA and the VSB need to be compared and be judged in consideration of the final free-field hearing threshold and speech discrimination in quiet and noise. In view of these requirements, the validity of some retrospective studies describing a better functional gain of VSB over CHA in the mid and high frequencies[30] must be critically questioned. Beltrame and colleagues[31] tried to evaluate the VSB gain in relation to patients' hearing needs by comparing the results with the individual average target gains provided by the customization algorithm of the National Acoustics Laboratories, Non-Linear, version 1 (NAL-NL1) and found that most patients failed to reach the predicted functional gains. In their study, speech reception in noise required a signal-to-noise ratio 7 to 13 dB greater than normal-hearing control subjects.

A fairly good attempt to compare VSB with CHA has been recently made by Marino and colleagues[33] who also used the NAL-NL1 prescription to optimize the CHA fitting before VSB implantation. Here, comparable speech test results were achieved with VSB and CHA in quiet, but VSB performance was substantially better in most speech-in-noise test conditions. Note that in this study 28% of the patients required revision surgery because of intermittent or no sound perception through the device and in two patients hearing remained unsatisfying despite revision surgery. Atas and colleagues[37] customized the preoperative fitting of CHA with the revised NAL regulations, but no audiometric data were reported and follow-up time was only 3 months.

In summary, the VSB at least provides hearing results that are similar to CHA, and may offer an advantage for speech-in-noise understanding.

CLINICAL RESULTS IN THE LITERATURE

Clinical results have been evaluated by using different questionnaires. Baumgartner and colleagues[8] used three different questionnaires in a multicenter study to assess subjective benefits of VSB patients. Compared with the unaided situation, they found significant improvement in most subtests evaluating different hearing situations, quality of life, and further social and physical aspects.

Using the International Outcome Inventory for Hearing Aids (IOI-HA) questionnaire Atas and colleagues[37] found the VSB in 19 patients with conductive or mixed hearing loss to be superior to CHA in two of seven items ("hearing benefit" and "residual participation restrictions") with the total score of the IOI-HA being significantly better for VSB than for CHA. With the same questionnaire, Hüttenbrink and colleagues[23] found four of seven items to be rated superior by patients with a clip vibroplasty, but instead of an inner-group preoperative-postoperative control they used a historical control group of CHA users. Yu and colleagues[36] had all seven questionnaire items of the IOI-HA to trend better by their eight patients with an RW-VSB, but statistical analysis failed to show a statistically significant difference.

Overall, most studies on VSB implantation for conductive or mixed hearing loss describe a remarkable subjective satisfaction among the implanted patients, an improvement in quality of life, with only minor impact on the aversiveness scale.[29] Among the audiologic criteria, patients mainly report a better sound quality, less feedback, and less occlusion with the VSB when compared with a CHA.[35]

REVISION SURGERY

Studies of the VSB have reported a revision surgery rate between 10% and 30%,[8,28,33] but in some studies information on this topic is missing.[31] The most common reason for revision surgery was insufficient hearing improvement, and thus a need for FMT repositioning.[29] Other long-term reasons to remove an implant include medically uncontrollable inflammation at the implant region or device failures, which might be related to head trauma.

SUMMARY

There is growing evidence for the effectiveness and safety of the VSB in patients with conductive and mixed hearing loss. The indications for implantation of a VSB are primarily related to intolerance of a CHA. A wide range of FMT coupling methods have been developed, which may result in similar acoustic outcomes. Complications are rare and are mainly related to insufficient functional hearing gain with the need to reposition the FMT in the RW niche. Studies indicate that the VSB can provide functional hearing gains at least as good as those achieved with CHA.

REFERENCES

1. Luers JC, Hüttenbrink K, Zahnert T, et al. Vibroplasty for mixed and conductive hearing loss. Otol Neurotol 2013;34:1005–12.

2. Ball GR. The Vibrant Soundbridge: design and development. In: Böheim K, editor. Active middle ear implants. Basel (Switzerland): Karger; 2010. p. 1–13.
3. Snik AF, Cremers CW. First audiometric results with the Vibrant Soundbridge, a semi-implantable hearing device for sensorineural hearing loss. Audiology 1999;38:335–8.
4. Tjellstrom A, Luetje CM, Hough JV, et al. Acute human trial of the floating mass transducer. Ear Nose Throat J 1997;76:204–6, 209–10.
5. Colletti V, Soli SD, Carner M, et al. Treatment of mixed hearing losses via implantation of a vibratory transducer on the round window. Int J Audiol 2006;45:600–8.
6. Verhaegen VJ, Mylanus EA, Cremers CW, et al. Audiological application criteria for implantable hearing aid devices: a clinical experience at the Nijmegen ORL clinic. Laryngoscope 2008;118:1645–9.
7. Verhaegen VJ, Mulder JJ, Cremers CW, et al. Application of active middle ear implants in patients with severe mixed hearing loss. Otol Neurotol 2012;33:297–301.
8. Baumgartner WD, Boheim K, Hagen R, et al. The vibrant soundbridge for conductive and mixed hearing losses: European multicenter study results. Adv Otorhinolaryngol 2010;69:38–50.
9. Cremers CW, O'Connor AF, Helms J, et al. International consensus on Vibrant Soundbridge(R) implantation in children and adolescents. Int J Pediatr Otorhinolaryngol 2010;74:1267–9.
10. Mandala M, Colletti L, Colletti V. Treatment of the atretic ear with round window vibrant soundbridge implantation in infants and children: electrocochleography and audiologic outcomes. Otol Neurotol 2011;32:1250–5.
11. Zernotti ME, Arauz SL, Di Gregorio MF, et al. Vibrant Soundbridge in congenital osseous atresia: multicenter study of 12 patients with osseous atresia. Acta Otolaryngol 2013;133:569–73.
12. Frenzel H, Hanke F, Beltrame M, et al. Application of the Vibrant Soundbridge to unilateral osseous atresia cases. Laryngoscope 2009;119:67–74.
13. Roman S, Denoyelle F, Farinetti A, et al. Middle ear implant in conductive and mixed congenital hearing loss in children. Int J Pediatr Otorhinolaryngol 2012;76:1775–8.
14. Verhaert N, Mojallal H, Schwab B. Indications and outcome of subtotal petrosectomy for active middle ear implants. Eur Arch Otorhinolaryngol 2013;270:1243–8.
15. Mlynski R, Mueller J, Hagen R. Surgical approaches to position the Vibrant Soundbridge in conductive and mixed hearing loss. Operative Techniques in Otolaryngology-Head and Neck Surgery 2010;21:272–7.
16. Kontorinis G, Lenarz T, Mojallal H, et al. Power stapes: an alternative method for treating hearing loss in osteogenesis imperfecta? Otol Neurotol 2011;32:589–95.
17. Wagner JH, Ernst A, Todt I. Magnet resonance imaging safety of the Vibrant Soundbridge system: a review. Otol Neurotol 2011;32:1040–6.
18. Vent J, Luers JC, Beutner D. Half-open bony channel technique for fixation of the Vibrant Soundbridge. Clin Otolaryngol 2009;34:87–8.
19. Beutner D, Helmstaedter V, Stumpf R, et al. The impact of partial mastoid obliteration on caloric vestibular function in canal wall-down mastoidectomy. Otol Neurotol 2010;31(9):1399–403.
20. Zahnert T, Hüttenbrink KB, Murbe D, et al. Experimental investigations of the use of cartilage in tympanic membrane reconstruction. Am J Otol 2000;21:322–8.
21. Roland PS, Wright CG, Isaacson B. Cochlear implant electrode insertion: the round window revisited. Laryngoscope 2007;117:1397–402.
22. Pennings RJ, Ho A, Brown J, et al. Analysis of Vibrant Soundbridge placement against the round window membrane in a human cadaveric temporal bone model. Otol Neurotol 2010;31:998–1003.

23. Hüttenbrink K, Beutner D, Bornitz M, et al. Clip vibroplasty: experimental evaluation and first clinical results. Otol Neurotol 2011;32:650–3.
24. Hüttenbrink KB, Zahnert T, Bornitz M, et al. TORP-vibroplasty: a new alternative for the chronically disabled middle ear. Otol Neurotol 2008;29:965–71.
25. Hüttenbrink KB, Beutner D, Zahnert T. Clinical results with an active middle ear implant in the oval window. Adv Otorhinolaryngol 2010;69:27–31.
26. Beutner D, Luers JC, Huttenbrink KB. Cartilage "shoe": a new technique for stabilisation of titanium total ossicular replacement prosthesis at centre of stapes footplate. J Laryngol Otol 2008;122:682–6.
27. Schwab B, Salcher RB, Maier H, et al. Oval window membrane vibroplasty for direct acoustic cochlear stimulation: treating severe mixed hearing loss in challenging middle ears. Otol Neurotol 2012;33:804–9.
28. Bernardeschi D, Hoffman C, Benchaa T, et al. Functional results of Vibrant Soundbridge middle ear implants in conductive and mixed hearing losses. Audiol Neurootol 2011;16:381–7.
29. Verhaert N, Desloovere C, Wouters J. Acoustic hearing implants for mixed hearing loss: a systematic review. Otol Neurotol 2013;34:1201–9.
30. Gunduz B, Atas A, Bayazit YA, et al. Functional outcomes of Vibrant Soundbridge applied on the middle ear windows in comparison with conventional hearing aids. Acta Otolaryngol 2012;132:1306–10.
31. Beltrame AM, Martini A, Prosser S, et al. Coupling the Vibrant Soundbridge to cochlea round window: auditory results in patients with mixed hearing loss. Otol Neurotol 2009;30:194–201.
32. Linder T, Schlegel C, DeMin N, et al. Active middle ear implants in patients undergoing subtotal petrosectomy: new application for the Vibrant Soundbridge device and its implication for lateral cranium base surgery. Otol Neurotol 2009;30:41–7.
33. Marino R, Linton N, Eikelboom RH, et al. A comparative study of hearing aids and round window application of the Vibrant Sound Bridge (VSB) for patients with mixed or conductive hearing loss. Int J Audiol 2013;52:209–18.
34. Colletti V, Carner M, Colletti L. TORP vs round window implant for hearing restoration of patients with extensive ossicular chain defect. Acta Otolaryngol 2009;129:449–52.
35. Tysome JR, Moorthy R, Lee A, et al. Systematic review of middle ear implants: do they improve hearing as much as conventional hearing aids? Otol Neurotol 2010;31(9):1369–75.
36. Yu JK, Tsang WS, Wong TK, et al. Outcome of Vibrant Soundbridge middle ear implant in Cantonese-speaking mixed hearing loss adults. Clin Exp Otorhinolaryngol 2012;5(Suppl 1):S82–8.
37. Atas A, Tutar H, Gunduz B, et al. Vibrant Sound Bridge application to middle ear windows versus conventional hearing aids: a comparative study based on international outcome inventory for hearing aids. Eur Arch Otorhinolaryngol 2014;271(1):35–40.

Vibrant Soundbridge Rehabilitation of Sensorineural Hearing Loss

Andleeb Khan, MD, Todd Hillman, MD, Douglas Chen, MD*

KEYWORDS

• Vibrant Soundbridge • Implantable middle ear devices • Sensorineural hearing loss

KEY POINTS

- The Vibrant Soundbridge is an option for amplification for patients with mild to severe sensorineural hearing loss.
- The device is most commonly placed through a mastoidectomy and facial recess approach. It is directly fixed to the incus to vibrate the ossicular chain.
- Overall, patients have increased functional gain and speech intelligibility and report better satisfaction compared with traditional amplification via hearing aids.

INTRODUCTION

For years, patients diagnosed with mild to severe sensorineural hearing loss were offered hearing aids as the best treatment. However, acoustic feedback and occlusion effect have frequently left many patients dissatisfied with amplification, despite advances in signal processing and device miniaturization. In 2000, the US Food and Drug Administration (FDA) approved the Vibrant Soundbridge (VSB), the first active implantable middle ear device available in the United States and Canada.[1] The commercial release of the device in Europe preceded this in February 1998.[2] The principle of middle ear implants is to bypass the tympanic membrane and impart mechanical vibrations directly to the ossicular chain to improve signal coupling.

The VSB device is a partially implanted electromagnetic device from Vibrant Med El (Med El Corporation, Innsbruck, Austria).[2] The VSB system consists of 2 parts that provide electromagnetic, direct-drive amplification when coupled. The first is an externally worn digital Audio Processor that picks up sound signal and amplifies it to a level appropriate for the sensorineural hearing loss. The earlier version of the processor, the AP 304, is no longer available. Its successor was the AP 404, which is now an alternative to the most current processor called the Amadé. Both of these processors are fully

Pittsburgh Ear Associates, Suite 402, 420 East North Avenue, Pittsburgh, PA 15212, USA
* Corresponding author.
E-mail address: Douglasachen@yahoo.com

Otolaryngol Clin N Am 47 (2014) 927–939
http://dx.doi.org/10.1016/j.otc.2014.08.005
0030-6665/14/$ – see front matter © 2014 Elsevier Inc. All rights reserved.

digital. The Amadé features output gain capability of up to 54 dB versus 45 dB of the AP 404. In addition, it has directional microphone capability as well as the option to select 1 of 3 programs most suitable to the listening environment. The amplified sound is then transmitted to the receiver coil of the second component, the implanted vibrating ossicular prosthesis (VORP). At the VORP's distal end is the floating mass transducer (FMT), which is fixed to the incus and directly drives it via mechanical motion (**Fig. 1**A).[3] The FMT comprises 2 electromagnetic coils sealed in a titanium housing that contains a magnet and is smaller than a grain of rice (see **Fig.** 1B). It is specifically designed to avoid mass-loading the ossicular chain.[1]

CANDIDACY FOR SURGERY

In the United States, The VSB System is indicated for adults 18 years and older who have moderate-to-severe sensorineural hearing loss that desire an alternative to an acoustic hearing aid.[4] European centers are implanting children older than 3 years of age.[5] Ideal candidates for middle ear implants are patients with high-frequency sensorineural hearing loss that have tried conventional amplification without success because of acoustic feedback, the occlusion effect, or inadequate high-frequency amplification. These limitations can be particularly pronounced in patients with good low-frequency hearing thresholds.[6] Although cochlear implants have been available for profound sensorineural hearing loss, otologists could offer only hearing aids to patients with moderate-to-severe sensorineural hearing loss. The VSB is a surgical solution for these patients. **Fig. 2** shows Med El Corporation's criteria for candidacy in patients with sensorineural hearing loss.

PREOPERATIVE PLANNING AND PREPARATION

It is important for both surgeon and audiologist to counsel the patient regarding the risks of surgery as well as the benefits and limitations of the device. Besides a history and physical examination, preoperative evaluation consists of a standard audiologic test battery, using a combination of aided and unaided conditions. These tests include tympanometry, acoustic reflex thresholds, pure-tone and bone-conduction thresholds as well as speech testing.[7] CT imaging is not mandatory but advisable. Facial nerve monitoring is especially useful in cases of congenital temporal bone anomalies or revision surgeries. Patients can undergo VSB implantation on an outpatient basis.

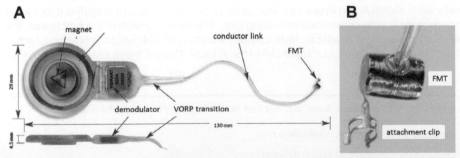

Fig. 1. (*A*) Components of the vibrating ossicular prosthesis (VORP). (*B*) Floating mass transducer (FMT). (*Courtesy of* MED-EL Corporation, Durham, NC; with permission.)

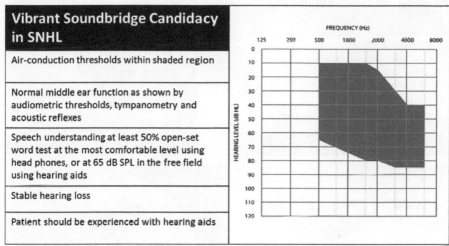

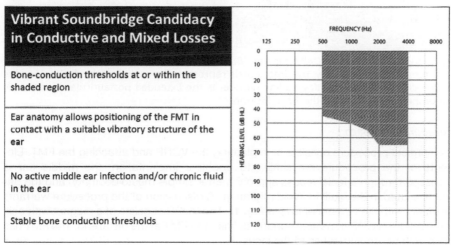

Fig. 2. (A) Vibrant Soundbridge candidacy in sensorineural hearing loss. (B) Vibrant Sound-bridge candidacy in conductive and mixed losses.

SURGICAL TECHNIQUE
Patient Preparation

The patient is positioned as is routine for otologic procedures. Preoperative sedative followed by anesthesia is administered and facial nerve monitoring electrodes are applied. The postauricular area is shaved and disinfected. A silicone VORP template oriented in a 45° posterosuperior axis is placed on the skin to determine optimal implant position (**Fig. 3**A). The VORP should not lie under the auricle, which can be ensured by marking the skull with methylene blue and placing the VORP posterior to this point. In addition, the VORP transition should sit at the posterior edge of the intended mastoidectomy (see **Fig. 3**B). The incision is marked on the skin and should be 2 cm from the edge of the template (see **Fig. 3**C, D).

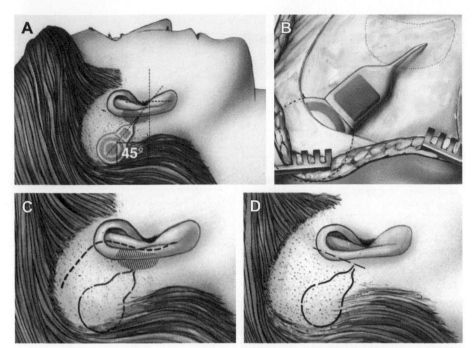

Fig. 3. (*A*) Orientation of VORP template. (*B*) The VORP transition at the posterior edge of the intended mastoidectomy. The dotted circle represents the outline of the device deep the temporalis muscle. (*C*) The dashed line represents the Extended postauricular incision. (*D*) The dashed line represents the Small incision.

Procedural Approach

The surgical procedure consists of implanting the VORP and attaching the FMT. Elements of the procedure are similar to cochlear implantation: the middle ear is accessed through a facial recess approach after simple mastoidectomy, and the device is seated in the skull to avoid migration. A discussion of the procedure warrants familiarity with the components (see **Fig. 1**). The VORP consists of a magnet with coil, demodulator, VORP transition, conductor link, and FMT at the distal end. The FMT has a clip with which it attaches to the incus.

After an incision is made, a pericranial flap is elevated. To ensure proper attachment of the magnet, the total thickness of the skin overlying the receiving coil should not exceed 7 mm. A portion of the pericranial flap can be excised to achieve the appropriate thickness, but care must be taken to have continuous fascial coverage over the demodulator, the transition, and the conductor link. A sterilized VORP template is placed on the skull to verify sufficient exposure.

Next, a simple mastoidectomy is performed to the point that the short process of the incus is visualized. Bony overhangs are left at the periphery to help with conductor link retention. A device seat is then drilled, which allows the transition of the conductor link to slope deeply in the mastoid cavity. The conductor link should be as medial to the skull surface as possible. The VORP template is positioned using the previously marked reference so that the critical positioning of the transition point is correct (**Fig. 4**). As in a cochlear implant, a channel is drilled from the seat to the mastoidectomy cavity for the VORP transition. Tie-down holes are created to fixate the demodulator (see **Fig. 4**).

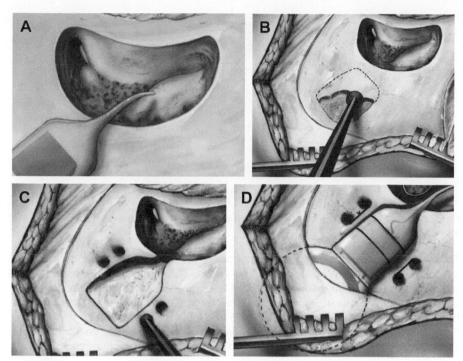

Fig. 4. (*A*) The transition point of the VORP at the posterior edge of the mastoidectomy. (*B*) A recess is drilled for the demodulator. (*C*) Tie-down holes to fix the VORP. (*D*) Positioned VORP. The dotted line represents the outline of the device deep to the temporalis muscle.

A facial recess is drilled and enlarged with inferior extension, to allow introduction of the FMT. A 2.5- to 3.0-mm burr approximates the size of the FMT and should pass through the recess as a test of adequate space. Care is taken to preserve the incus buttress so that the ligament attached to the short process is not violated.

The VORP is introduced into the field, at which point monopolar cautery is no longer used. It is positioned so that the FMT lies in the mastoidectomy defect. The demodulator is sutured in place. The FMT is then advanced through the mastoidectomy and positioned so that its clip is over the superior portion of the incus long process. The axis of the FMT should be parallel to the axis of motion of the stapes and must be in intimate contact with the incudostapedial joint (**Fig. 5**). Special forceps (**Fig. 6**) are used to close the clip to encircle the incus. At this point, if the attachment is too loose, the clip can be tightened with fine alligator forceps. An alternative method advocated by the senior author is to elevate a tympanomeatal flap to augment exposure for tightening because this is difficult even through a widened facial recess.

The conductor link is then arranged so that there is slack at the FMT, and so that it does not contact the walls of the facial recess. In the mastoidectomy, it is tucked under the bony overhangs. The FMT position is then once again confirmed under magnification. It should not contact the promontory, tympanic membrane, or pyramidal eminence. The final position of the FMT is demonstrated in **Fig. 6**. The pericranial flap is sutured over the anterior portion of the demodulator, the transition, and conductor link. The skin flap is then closed in 2 layers.[7]

Some authors have described what has been called a transcanal approach, whereby a very small partial mastoidectomy is created to accommodate the coil of the device.

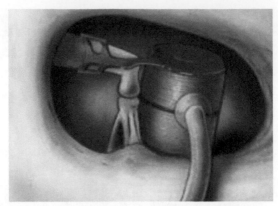

Fig. 5. The FMT is in contact with the incudostapedial joint and stapes, parallel to its axis of motion.

To gain access to the middle ear, the posterior bony canal is slightly widened so that the structures of the mesotympanum become visible. This widening can be augmented with a superior atticotomy to expose more of the long process of the incus and the incudostapedial joint. A modification as a result of this approach through the external auditory canal is that the clip must be rotated 45 to 90° to facilitate clipping onto the incus. Purported advantages include less operative time by avoiding mastoidectomy, greater ease in introducing the bulky FMT into the middle ear, and easier crimping.[8,9]

POTENTIAL COMPLICATIONS AND MANAGEMENT OF THESE COMPLICATIONS

The conductor link and FMT are fragile and should only be handled by the surgeon. As such, repeated manipulation of the FMT attachment including grasping it at its junction to the wire is discouraged to avoid damage to the device. The conductor link has the potential to impede the movement of the FMT if it contacts the bony walls of the facial recess but can be avoided by prebending a small curve in the conductor link so that it clears the wall. An additional concern regarding the conductor link is the possibility of extrusion through the skin, either with suboptimal placement in the mastoid or with the transcanal approaches, where its position lies closer to the skin surface.

Although the placement of the VORP and FMT is crucial to appropriate device function, it is important to ensure a thin enough flap for the external audio processor to attach to the VORP's magnet. A skin flap gauge can be used to check the thickness. Temporalis muscle can be resected to thin the flap. If additional thinning is required, the skin flap should not be thinned enough to expose hair follicles.

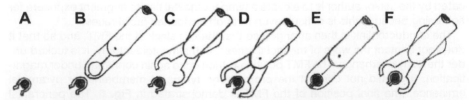

Fig. 6. Forming forceps with cross-section of long process of the incus. (A) The clip in position on the long process of the incus. (B) The forming forceps advanced with the jaws closed. (C) The jaws opened. (D) The forceps advanced over the attachment. (E) The jaws closed causing the clip to encircle the incus. (F) The jaws opened and the forceps removed.

Erosion of the long process of the incus may be a potential long-term problem, although Todt and colleagues[10] report a microscopic examination of an incus after 4 years of FMT clamp fixation that demonstrated histologic findings similar to those after stapes surgery, likely due to the up and down movement of the FMT's titanium clamp with vibration. The attachment is firm but not completely sealed, due to the inherent properties of titanium compared with other materials.

Facial nerve paralysis is a risk for any operation requiring a facial recess approach, and in theory, particularly for implantation of the VSB because such a large facial recess is required. Despite the need for a larger facial recess, facial paralysis has not been reported in the literature to date. Another consequence of having to extend the facial recess dissection is the risk of damage to the chorda tympani nerve. Unlike facial nerve injury, this complication has been reported. In a multicenter study of 125 patients, a rate of self-reported taste disturbance at long-term follow-up was reported at 6.5%.[11]

POSTPROCEDURAL CARE
Medical Follow-up and Audiology Follow-up

Eight weeks after surgery, the patient returns for clearance by the surgeon to have the audiologist dispense and activate the Audio Processor. After initial VSB fitting, follow up assessments for reprogramming are offered at several intervals. In the authors' practice, these follow-up assessments were at 1, 3, 6, and 10 months, although many patients were satisfied after the first visit and did not require further program adjustments.

Rehabilitation and Recovery

The VSB has a magnet for the fixation of the Audio Processor, which is not removable, similar to cochlear implant technology. Unlike a cochlear implant, the VSB has an additional magnetic component (ie, the FMT) fixed to the incus by a titanium clamp. MRI scanning has been known to demagnetize cochlear implant devices. For the VSB, magnetic forces could dislocate the FMT and/or impair the ossicular chain, or produce noise trauma. As such, the manufacturer suggests MRI scanning would be contraindicated and may impair the function and integrity of the device. MRI scanning at 1.5 T of 2 patients implanted with the VSB has been reported, without any compromise of functional integrity and without any fractures of the skull surface.[10] A case of revision surgery has also been reported after MRI imaging caused displacement of the implant.[11]

Monopolar cautery is not to be used during future surgical procedures per the manufacturer's formal recommendation. Electrosurgical instruments are capable of producing radiofrequency voltages that can directly interact with the implant. The induced currents can cause damage to the implant and to the patient's hearing. In these surgical cases, alternatives such as bipolar cautery or ultrasonic (harmonic) scalpel should be first alternatives, although it should be noted that cochlear implants have the same theoretic concerns, but monopolar cautery has been used with little difficulty for surgery below the clavicles. Furthermore, due to very high electrical currents applied to the head, electroconvulsive therapy is contraindicated in patients with the VSB.

The effect of imaging studies such as PET scans and linear acceleration techniques are unknown. Patients are instructed to exercise water precautions while wearing the Audio Processor.

SURGICAL AND HEARING OUTCOMES

Measurements on temporal bones have shown the VSB to produce maximum output comparable to sounds of approximately 110 dB SPL.[12] In 1998, Snik and Cremers[13] reported the first audiometric results with the VSB in a series of 7 patients. Increased gain was demonstrated for soft sounds and moderate sounds (21 and 17 dB, respectively). Speech recognition tests were also evaluated and demonstrated speech gain ranging from 13 to 28 dB. Smaller gain at higher input levels was observed, reflecting the nonlinear amplification of the VSB. Although sound processors were adjusted to maximal gain, a range of gain values was seen at any given input level, suggesting factors other than the processor parameters determine gain. The authors surmised this could perhaps be due to the tightness of the transducer-incus coupling. Nonetheless, this preliminary data were very promising for the use of VSB in hearing-impaired patients who could not tolerate ear molds.

Snik and Cremers[13] further reported on a series of 5 patients wherein the presence of the transducer did not have any effect on the air-conduction thresholds. Interestingly, the bone-conduction thresholds at 0.5 and 1 kHz improved, thought to be due to the addition of mass to the middle ear structures, which has been demonstrated to improve hearing via bone conduction in the low-frequency range.

Surgical outcomes were first reported in 2001, in a multicenter study in France on 25 patients.[14] In 19 of 25 patients, the authors reported surgery as being uneventful. In the remaining 6 patients, challenges were encountered with either a facial recess that was too small to introduce the forming forceps or a suboptimal fixation of the clip due to the small diameter of the incus long process. One patient experienced the adverse event of transient facial paresis occurring 10 days after surgery and resolving after 6 weeks. Three patients reported pain over the implant site that resolved several months after surgery, possibly related to the use of an enlarged retro-auricular incision. No change in residual postoperative hearing was noted in this patient series. Functional gain was significantly superior with the VSB, particularly with the use of the Vibrant D digital processor compared with the older analog version, the Vibrant P, and compared with preoperative hearing aids. Despite objective speech testing showing no significant difference, 70% of patients reported decreased difficulty with hearing in environments with competing background noise. Although most (76%) patients wore the VSB alone, some patients chose to resume their contralateral hearing aid because of the severity of their bilateral hearing loss.

An FDA phase III clinical trial reported on 53 adults implanted with the VSB for sensorineural hearing loss, and patients were followed for a period of 5 months after surgery.[4] Safety of the VSB was demonstrated with confirmation that there was no significant difference in mean residual hearing thresholds and immittance measures after activation of the device. Ninety-eight percent of patients had tympanometry results consistent with normal middle ear pressure and compliance, and there was no change in the presence of acoustic reflexes. Efficacy was demonstrated by functional gain, word recognition, and self-assessment. This study measured a mean 14.1-dB gain ($P<.001$) with the use of the Vibrant D processor. Speech recognition was evaluated more rigorously than previous studies. Aided word-recognition in quiet showed no difference compared with presurgery hearing aids, as was seen in an earlier study. However, unlike the prior study, speech recognition in the presence of background noise was found to increase by an average of 6% with the Vibrant D processor compared with the aided presurgery condition with conventional amplification. Again, no improvement was seen with the older Vibrant P processor. Although 6% may seem a modest figure, the authors report scores on the Revised Speech Perception in Noise test with the Vibrant D processor group improved over the preoperative unaided condition by a factor of 5 and over the presurgery acoustic hearing aid by a factor of 4. Of note, measures were taken to standardize the presurgery aided condition: aids were appropriately fit based on a standardized procedure (the National Acoustic

Laboratories-Revised [NAL-R]), and word recognition score was at least 50%. In addition, patients with abnormal middle ear anatomy and retrocochlear loss were excluded.

Finally, patients in this series completed several detailed inventories. Compared with presurgery-aided conditions, the number of subjects who reported improvement was significant across 7 subscales of the Profile of Hearing Aid Performance, including reduced cues, reverberation, and distortion of sounds. On the Hearing Device Satisfaction Scale, 94% rated overall improvement of "overall sound quality," 88% improved their satisfaction rate with "effectiveness in background noise," and 98% expressed satisfaction with "overall fit and comfort." Questionnaires also assessed device performance in specific situations. Most were best able to understand speech with the VSB in all situations except for using the telephone, although this may not have been a fair representation because the worse ear (and thus the ear not used for the telephone) was chosen for implantation. The strongest preference for the device was "one-to-one conversations" (76%), while the lowest was at "live performance at theaters" (53%). Results of these questionnaires can guide surgeons during preoperative counseling, as patients may relate more to satisfaction results in particular situations as it relates to their daily lives, rather than data regarding functional gain.

The largest VSB surgical series, to date, is a French multicenter study of 125 patients.[2] Hearing outcomes paralleled those of prior studies in terms of no change in residual postoperative hearing. Gain was found to correlate with the degree of hearing loss (ie, steady increase in gain as degree of hearing loss increased) for 0.5, 1, and 2 kHz. In contrast, mean functional gain remained fairly constant at 4 kHz irrespective of degree of hearing loss. Although previous data suggested no improvement of speech recognition in quiet with the VSB, findings in this study demonstrated otherwise. Most patients were globally satisfied per standardized and nonstandardized assessments (83% and 89%, respectively). No correlation was observed between satisfaction ratings and objective outcome measures, suggesting test data alone do not fully reflect the success of treatment.

This series was also the first to report intraoperative events in 17 of 125 surgeries (**Table 1**).

The most commonly encountered incident was narrow diameter of the incus (8 cases), followed by restricted facial recess (5 cases). Chorda tympani was severed in 2 cases, and the forming forceps malfunctioned in one surgery. No serious events, such as facial nerve injury or disruption of the ossicular chain, were reported. Five cases of device malfunction were seen in follow-up and were subsequently explanted, and all of these malfunctions were attributed to an earlier version of the device

Table 1
Intraoperative incidents

	Reportable Incidents for 125 Surgeries from the Surgeon Survey				
Incident	Narrow Incus Diameter	Restricted Posterior-Tympanotomy	Severed Chorda Tympanii	Restricted Mastoid Space	Forceps Malfunction
Subtotal	8	5	2	1	1
Incident rate (%)	6.4	4	1.6	0.8	0.8

From Sterkers O, Boucarra D, Labassi S, et al. A middle ear implant, the Symphonix Vibrant Soundbridge: retrospective study of the first 125 patients implanted in France. Otol Neurotol 2003;24(3):429; with permission.

manufactured before May 1999.[15] The present failure rate for devices made after this date is reported as 0.03%. The most common adverse symptoms reported following VSB implant surgery is aural fullness, followed by taste disturbance (**Table 2**). Both of these resolve in roughly half of the patients.[16]

Aside from histologic modification of the incus caused by FMT fixation, potential long-term side effects have been postulated to occur as a consequence of cochlear trauma due to overstimulation of the ossicular chain. Assessment over a period of 2 years postimplant of a series of 20 patients is reported by Schmuziger and colleagues.[16] These findings were somewhat contrary to outcomes measured by previous VSB studies. Residual hearing in the implanted ear was poorer by a mean threshold elevation of 8 dB. This study found aided speech perception in noise was comparable between the VSB and hearing aids worn before surgery, and that speech perception in silence was actually better with hearing aids. Patients were still globally satisfied with the VSB by subjective measures despite rating perceived speech benefit lower than cosmetic results, sound quality, and comfort. Three of 20 patients had persistent taste alterations, and pooled results from prior studies indicate an overall rate of 6% long-term chorda tympani–related taste disturbance.

Long-term shifts in postoperative hearing thresholds were corroborated in a series of 39 patients, 25 of whom had follow-up of greater than 1 year.[15] Threshold changes were stratified by frequency, with a significant change in hearing thresholds over time at 0.5 kHz (2.79 dB, $P = .008$) and 4 kHz (3.34 dB, $P = .002$). However, this was not statistically significant compared with the contralateral ear. Thresholds at 1 and 2 kHz remained stable. A plausible explanation for this observed threshold shift is because of the mass loading of the FMT on the incudostapedial joint and stapes. Studies have been conducted on mass-loaded ossicular chains and have shown threshold modifications particularly in the high frequencies. As the load on the stapes increases, auditory response as measured by auditory-evoked potentials decreases at high frequencies. Cadaveric studies have shown that the greater the mass, the less stapes displacement, and this occurred at all frequencies.

As multiple studies have indicated, patients have been satisfied overall with their quality of life after VSB implantation. As such, a subset of patients has requested a second implant to further improve gain. The effect of bilateral implantation has been

Table 2
Side effects from VSB implantation

	Patient-Reported Side Effects (N = 95)	
Side Effect	Frequency Reported (% Total)	Long-term Side Effect (% Total)
Fullness	20.0	9.7
Taste disturbance	13.7	6.5
Vertigo	11.7	0
Decreased hearing	8.5	3.2
Pain	7.4	1.1
Headache	4.2	0
Infection	3.9	0
Other (eg, tinnitus)	3.2	1.1

From Sterkers O, Boucarra D, Labassi S, et al. A middle ear implant, the Symphonix Vibrant Soundbridge: retrospective study of the first 125 patients implanted in France. Otol Neurotol 2003;24(3):432; with permission.

examined by Garin and colleagues.[17] The advantages of binaural amplification over unilateral amplification are well known, and these include better speech understanding in noisy environments and better sound localization and sound quality. Fifteen patients with symmetric sensorineural hearing loss were evaluated for functional gain, speech intelligibility, and subjective benefits. Maximum gain with bilateral VSB implantation was 36 dB at 2 kHz. Word recognition in noise was best when the patients were tested with the VSB implant in both ears compared with testing in the unilateral VSB condition for the right and left ear. In quiet, at lower presentation levels (40 dB), bilateral amplification also improved word recognition. No benefits of binaural amplification were seen at higher intensity levels because of a ceiling effect on speech intelligibility, although other authors have found statistically significant improvement in speech recognition threshold in quiet with bilateral VSB.[18] In terms of general satisfaction, patients were found to be very satisfied after the first implant, but no further improvement in general satisfaction was obtained after adding a second VSB implant. Questions concerning particular listening aspects yielded higher scores for the bilateral VSB condition, particularly for the "ability to follow a conversation with several persons." The authors also questioned patients about complaints with the VSB. Two patients reported "distortion of loud sound"; 1 reported "metallic sound"; another reported "itching," and 1 patient thought the VSB was "too visible." Despite these reports, the main complaints about hearing aids (whistling due to feedback, annoyance of having a device in the ear, and poor sound quality) were all eliminated.

More recent data consist of several comparative studies between the VSB and hearing aids. Open fit hearing aids were specifically designed to benefit patients with high-frequency sensorineural hearing loss by leaving the ear unoccluded with little chance of acoustic feedback. Manufacturers of open fit hearing aids provide recommended hearing threshold indication fields to guide practitioners for appropriate patient selection. As with open fit hearing aids, recommended threshold fields are provided for the VSB as well. Because both are options for patients with high-frequency

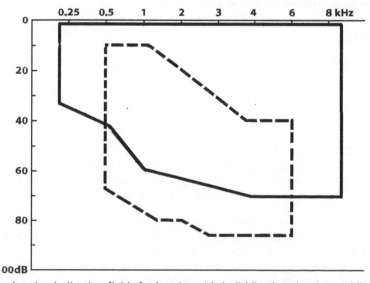

Fig. 7. Overlapping indication fields for hearing aids (*solid lines*) and active middle ear implants (*dashed lines*). (*Adapted from* Boeheim K, Pok SM, Schloegel M, et al. Active middle ear implant compared with open-fit hearing aid in sloping high-frequency sensorineural hearing loss. Otol Neurotol 2010;31(3):425; with permission.)

sensorineural hearing loss, there is significant overlap in the indication (**Fig. 7**). As such, outcome measures of the VSB versus an open fit hearing aid have been examined. In quiet, 50% speech comprehension is achieved at a significantly softer presentation level (4.7 dB, $P = .027$) with the VSB than with the SINGIA hearing aid (Siemens, Piscataway, New Jersey). The result was similar in noise (4.4 dB softer with the VSB, $P = .028$).[8] Other studies confirm superiority of the VSB to open fit hearing aids at high frequencies.[19]

REVISION SURGERY

Revision surgery most commonly occurs for device failures, as noted above. The literature also reports revision procedures for a case of a postoperative hematoma and for dislocation of the transducer after MRI imaging. In addition, there was an event related to confusion regarding the orientation of the VORP, which was placed with the incorrect side facing upwards. Because this reversed the polarity of the magnet, revision was required.[15] Although incus erosion has not yet been a problem in the author's experience, if this were to occur, the FMT would have to be placed in the round window niche.

SUMMARY

Among the active middle ear implants that are available today, the VSB is an effective alternative for rehabilitation of patients with high-frequency sensorineural hearing loss. Tests of subjective benefit of the VSB, either alone or in comparison with open-fit hearing aids, demonstrate patient satisfaction with the sound quality it provides. Audiologic data demonstrate increased gain and suggest that the VSB improves speech intelligibility. Although there is a dearth of long-term results and some divergence among results in audiologic outcomes, the VSB is a reasonable option for patients who seek an alternative to hearing aids.

REFERENCES

1. Ashburn-Reed S. The first FDA-approved middle ear implant: the Vibrant Soundbridge. Hear J 2001;54(8):47–8.
2. Sterkers O, Boucarra D, Labassi S, et al. A middle ear implant, the Symphonix Vibrant Soundbridge: retrospective study of the first 125 patients implanted in France. Otol Neurotol 2003;24(3):427–36.
3. Ball G. No more laughing at the deaf boy. Vienna (Austria): Haymon Verlag; 2011.
4. Luetje CM, Brackman D, Balkany T, et al. Phase III clinical trial results with the Vibrant Soundbridge implantable middle ear hearing device: a prospective controlled multicenter study. Otolaryngol Head Neck Surg 2002;126(2):97–107.
5. Med El Website Candidacy. Available at: http://www.medel.com/products-vsb-candidacy/.
6. Uziel A, Mondain M, Hagen P, et al. Rehabilitation for high-frequency sensorineural hearing impairment in adults with the Symphonix Vibrant Soundbridge: a comparative study. Otol Neurotol 2003;24(5):775–83.
7. Vibrant Soundbridge; The Implantable Hearing System Surgical guide, Med El. Available at: http://www.medel.com/data/pdf/28031.pdf.
8. Bruschini L, Forli F, Giannarelli M, et al. Exclusive transcanal surgical approach for Vibrant Soundbridge implantation: surgical and functional results. Otol Neurotol 2009;30(7):950–5.

9. Truy E, Eshraghi A, Balkany T, et al. Vibrant Soundbridge surgery: evaluation of transcanal surgical approaches. Otol Neurotol 2006;27(6):887–95.
10. Todt I, Seidl R, Mutze S, et al. MRI scanning and incus fixation in Vibrant Soundbridge implantation. Otol Neurotol 2004;25(6):969–72.
11. Fisch U, Cremers C, Lenarz T, et al. Clinical experience with the Vibrant Soundbridge implant device. Otol Neurotol 2001;6:962–72.
12. Snik AF, Mylanus EA, Cremers CW. Implantable hearing devices for sensorineural hearing loss: a review of the audiometric data. Clin Otolaryngol Allied Sci 1998; 23(5):414–9.
13. Snik FM, Cremers WR. First audiometric results with the Vibrant Soundbridge, a semi-implantable hearing device for sensorineural hearing loss. Int J Audiol 1999; 38(6):335–8.
14. Fraysse B, Lavieille J, Schmerber S, et al. A multicenter study of the Vibrant Soundbridge middle ear implant: early clinical results and experience. Otol Neurotol 2001;22(6):952–61.
15. Vincent C, Fraysse B, Lavieille J, et al. A longitudinal study on postoperative hearing thresholds with the Vibrant Soundbridge device. Eur Arch Otorhinolaryngol 2004;261(9):493–6.
16. Schmuziger N, Schimmann F, Wengen D, et al. Long-term assessment after implantation of the Vibrant Soundbridge device. Otol Neurotol 2006;27(2):183–8.
17. Garin P, Schmerber S, Magnan J, et al. Bilateral vibrant Soundbridge implantation: audiologic and subjective benefits in quiet and noisy environments. Acta Otolaryngol 2010;130(12):1370–8.
18. Saliba I, Calmels MN, Wanna G, et al. Binaurality in middle ear implant recipients using contralateral digital hearing aids. Otol Neurotol 2005;26:680–5.
19. Sziklai I, Szilvássy J. Functional gain and speech understanding obtained by Vibrant Soundbridge or by open-fit hearing aid. Acta Otolaryngol 2011;131(4): 428–33.

The Envoy Esteem Implantable Hearing System

Sam J. Marzo, MD[a],*, Joshua M. Sappington, MD[a],
Jack A. Shohet, MD[b]

KEYWORDS

- Envoy Esteem • Middle ear implantation • Implantable hearing aid
- Sensorineural hearing loss

KEY POINTS

- The Envoy Esteem is the first completely implantable hearing device.
- The Envoy Esteem is indicated for patients older than 18 years of age with stable moderate to severe sensorineural hearing loss and word discrimination scores greater than 40%.
- Patients undergoing implantation should have limited hearing benefit with best-fit hearing aids.
- The surgical procedure is technically demanding, and the best hearing results are typically seen at 6 months postoperatively.
- Complications with the Envoy Esteem are uncommon, and hearing is generally better than with hearing aids.

Videos of diode laser using to section incus long process, laser char removal from incus long process, completion of incus sectioning, cleaning of methylene blue from stapes capitulum, application of precoat to stapes capitulum, and application of cement around sensor and drive bodies accompany this article at http://www.oto.theclinics.com/

INTRODUCTION

Hearing loss is the number one sensory impairment and is a growing epidemic in the United States.[1] Hearing loss is generally classified as conductive, sensorineural, or mixed. Of these, sensorineural hearing loss is the most common. Approximately 11.3% of the United States population or 34.25 million people have hearing loss.

[a] Department of Otolaryngology-Head and Neck Surgery, Loyola University Medical Center, 2160 South First Avenue, Maywood, IL 60153, USA; [b] Shohet Ear Associates, New Port Beach, CA, USA
* Corresponding author.
E-mail address: smarzo@lumc.edu

Otolaryngol Clin N Am 47 (2014) 941–952
http://dx.doi.org/10.1016/j.otc.2014.08.006
0030-6665/14/$ – see front matter © 2014 Elsevier Inc. All rights reserved.

oto.theclinics.com

According to the National Institute on Deafness and Other Communication Disorders, approximately 17% of American adults report some degree of hearing loss.[1] It increases in all populations with age and is showing an alarming increase in adolescents.[2]

Approximately 8.5 million people wear hearing aids, but only 20% to 25% of individuals who could benefit from hearing aids actually wear them, for several reasons.[3] Financial considerations are undoubtedly important; hearing aids typically cost $1000 to $3000 each, with most patients requiring 2, and need to be replaced/upgraded on average every 5 years. Some patients do not like the appearance of hearing aids. Other people do not believe they have a hearing handicap, and some think their family members are pressuring them to obtain hearing aids.

Although many patients with hearing aids are satisfied with them, some complain of ear canal irritation, ear canal infections, feedback, and an occlusion effect. Hearing aids can break or can be lost. Most patients remove their hearing aids when they go to bed, thus requiring other assistive devices to hear appliances such as alarms and the phone. Furthermore, hearing aid batteries need to be replaced weekly, and the aids themselves have a limited lifespan of approximately 5 years before they need to be replaced.

Patients with mild to moderate hearing losses and good word discrimination, in general, do best with hearing aids. Patients with severe and profound hearing losses with poor word discrimination are better served with cochlear implants. Patients in the middle of these 2 groups (moderate to severe sensorineural hearing loss with word recognition scores greater than 40% while wearing hearing aids) are candidates for active middle ear implants, such as the Envoy Esteem.

DEVICE DESCRIPTION

The Envoy Esteem implantable hearing system is composed of a sound processor/battery, sensor, and driver. The sensor and driver are placed in the mastoid cavity (**Fig. 1**), whereas the sound processor/battery is placed in a subcutaneous pocket posterior to the mastoid cavity. The sensor is attached to the incus body. Movements of the tympanic membrane are transmitted to the malleus and incus. Through sensing vibrations of the incus, the sensor basically acts as an internal microphone. It sends electrical information via insulated wires to the replaceable/programmable sound processor/battery. From here, information is related to the driver, which is a piezoelectric

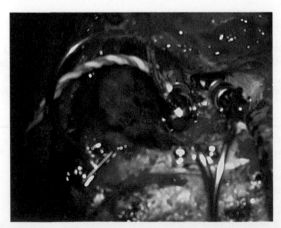

Fig. 1. Right mastoid cavity, with sensor seen on the left and driver seen on the right.

transducer attached to the stapes head. The stapes is then mechanically moved, which stimulates the cochlea. Through driving the ossicular chain directly, this middle ear implant can bypass some of the problems of conventional hearing aids.[4,5]

CANDIDACY FOR SURGERY

Patients who are candidates for the Envoy Esteem should be older than 18 years and have a stable moderate to severe sensorineural hearing loss with word recognition scores greater than 40%. Ideal candidates are those who have tried properly fitted hearing aids for at least 6 months. Because few if any insurance companies cover the procedure (which can range from $35,000–$45,000 per ear), patients should have sufficient finances so that the procedure would not cause excessive financial strain. Patients should also be in adequate health and be able to tolerate a general anesthetic.

Contraindications to surgery include a history of active chronic otitis media, cholesteatoma, otosclerosis, retrocochlear disease, inner ear malformations, documented fluctuating hearing loss, Meniere disease, otitis externa, disabling tinnitus, conductive or mixed hearing loss, and previous ossiculoplasty or stapes surgery. Patients who have undergone prior tympanostomy with pressure equalization tube placement and/or tympanoplasty might be candidates provided they do not have any residual conductive hearing loss. Other contraindications are the need for periodic MRI, because the device is not MRI-compatible; the presence of wound healing issues; and a history of prior radiotherapy to the ear and temporal bone.

PREOPERATIVE PLANNING AND PREPARATION

An important aspect in counseling patients about the Envoy Esteem is ensuring that patients have realistic expectations about the device. Not all patients will have the same or an ideal result with the device. The device may not overcome all of the limitations of their hearing aids, and the hearing may not be significantly better than that experienced with a pair of well-fit hearing aids. Furthermore, in many patients, the hearing slowly improves over several months after surgery, and several fittings/adjustments are necessary. For most patients, 2 to 3 device adjustments within the first 6 months are necessary. Revision surgery and/or explantation also may be necessary if the device is not functioning adequately or if surgical complications occur. Lastly, the patient will still likely require a hearing aid in the contralateral ear.

A 2004 phase I clinical trial reported on 57 patients with adverse events, including taste disturbance (40%), ear effusion (30%), and tinnitus (14%), and 3 patients (5%) required surgical revision.[4,6] Therefore, informed consent requires discussing potential intraoperative and postoperative complications, including the possibility of aborted surgery because of inadequate ossicular chain mobility, or inadequate space in the mastoid cavity. Other potential complications include bleeding, infection, tympanic membrane perforation, facial paresis or paralysis, deafness, vertigo, new or worsened tinnitus, injury to the ear canal, injury to the labyrinth, injury to the sigmoid sinus, and injury to the dura resulting in a cerebrospinal fluid leakage. Most patients will have a temporary ipsilateral taste disturbance because of sacrifice of the chorda tympani nerve, which is required in almost all cases.

Late complications can occur, and these most commonly include limited gain, feedback, scar tissue formation, worsened hearing, infection, biofilm formation, device exposure, and device extrusion. Revision surgery and/or device explantation may be necessary in selected cases. Although reconstruction of the ossicular chain can occur during explantation, the hearing results may not be the same as at baseline before implantation.

If a patient is deemed to be a good candidate for surgery and is interested in proceeding, a computed tomography (CT) scan of the temporal bones without contrast is obtained to ascertain if enough space is available for the sensor and driver. The distance between the stapes head and sigmoid sinus should be more than 22.0 mm, and the distance between the incus body and middle cranial fossa dural plate should be more than 2.5 mm. In patients with symmetric hearing between each ear, the larger mastoid is generally selected as the best ear to implant first.

SURGICAL TECHNIQUE
Patient Positioning

The patient is brought to the operating room and is placed on a padded operating table in the supine position. General anesthesia is administered via laryngotracheal intubation. A laryngeal mask airway is not recommended, because the total surgical time is approximately 3.5 hours. A short-acting paralytic anesthetic is administered, because facial nerve monitoring is used during the procedure. The table is turned 180°. The head is placed on a foam headrest and rotated away so that the operative ear is facing upward and taped in place. The facial nerve monitor electrodes are placed in the orbicularis oris and orbicularis oculi muscles and the monitor is tested to ensure it is working correctly.

Procedural Approach

The ideal sound processor location is marked on a flat part of the skull posterior to the anticipated mastoidectomy. An S-shaped incision is marked on the skin above and anterior to the anticipated sound processor position, curving toward the mastoid tip (**Fig. 2**). A small hair shave around the incision is performed. Plastic drapes are placed to protect the hair from blood and debris. Local anesthetic is infiltrated into the intended incision for hemostasis.

The incision and ear are prepared and draped in a sterile fashion. Using microscopic visualization, the ear canal is cleaned and a microphone is placed in the ear canal (**Fig. 3**) and checked to ensure it is working correctly. Because of the significant amount of intraoperative testing necessary to confirm correct device placement and

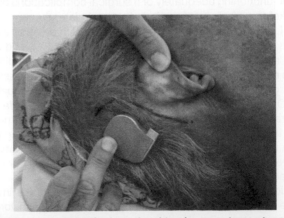

Fig. 2. An S-shaped incision is marked on the skin above and anterior to the anticipated sound processor position, curving toward the mastoid tip.

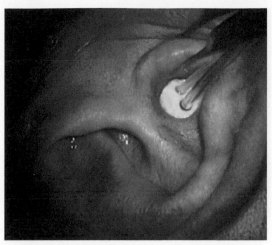

Fig. 3. Microphone in ear canal.

function, an Envoy company engineer familiar with the testing procedures should be present. The pinna is draped forward over the microphone and taped in place with a water-tight drape. The incision is made with a scalpel and anterior and posterior flaps are created. A stepped musculoperiosteal incision is made and the soft tissues are elevated off of the mastoid cortex.

A sound processor bed is drilled posterior to the mastoid cavity (**Fig. 4**). Using microdissection, an intact canal wall tympanomastoidectomy is performed. The bony external auditory canal is skeletonized. The epitympanum is drilled until the incus and head of the malleus are exposed. A wide facial recess approach is performed (**Fig. 5**). The chorda tympani nerve is resected and the facial recess is extended until the annulus is identified. The middle ear and mastoid are carefully irrigated to remove any bone dust, and hemostasis is obtained. Bone wax is not used, because the hydroxyapatite cement used to secure the sensor and driver in place will not adhere to it.

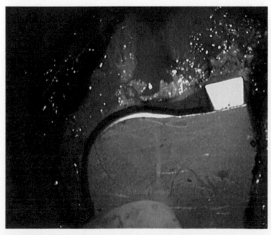

Fig. 4. Drilled sound processor bed for a right Envoy Esteem.

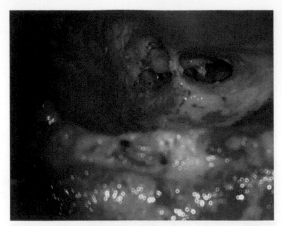

Fig. 5. Right intact canal wall tympanomastoidectomy with wide facial recess approach.

Any adhesions around the incus body and long process and the stapes superstructure are removed. A 0.3- to 0.4-mm piece of reflector tape is placed on the incus body and posterior crus of the stapes. The mobility of the incus and stapes are measured using laser Doppler vibrometry (**Fig. 6**).[7] This is done to ensure that there is adequate movement of the ossicles before implantation. The microphone in the ear produces a 100-dB noise across 50 frequencies ranging from 125 to 8000 Hz. The average movement of the incus and stapes is approximately 100 nm. Hypomobility of either the incus or stapes that cannot be corrected with adhesion removal will require aborting the surgical procedure at this point. Because the ossicular chain has not been disrupted, the hearing should be similar to baseline.

If the ossicular chain mobility is normal then the procedure can continue. Using a sharp knife such as a 59 blade, the incudostapedial joint is incised in a 360° fashion and the mucosa overlying the stapes head is reflected inferiorly. Moist Gelfoam is placed in the middle ear, protecting the tympanic segment of the facial nerve. Using a diode laser, the distal 3 to 4 mm of the incus long process (Video 1) is resected by cutting a deep grove. Because the laser will not cut through the black carbon

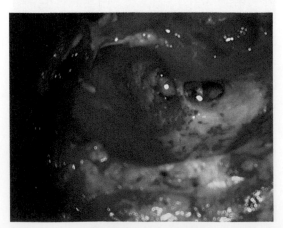

Fig. 6. The mobility of the incus and stapes are measured using laser Doppler vibrometry.

eschar that develops on the incus, this must be carefully picked away without dislocating the incus (Video 2). Keeping the Gelfoam moist while using the laser can prevent a heat injury to the facial nerve.

The incus long process is removed along with the Gelfoam (Video 3). The mucosa covering the stapes head is painted with methylene blue placed on a small piece of Gelfoam. The stapes head and neck are carefully cleaned, removing all of the stained mucosa (Video 4). This part of the procedure is very important for proper cement bonding. Once the stapes head is cleaned, it is dried with the laser. A small precoat of ionomeric cement is placed on the stapes head and neck and allowed to dry (Video 5).

Next, stabilizer bars are screwed into the mastoid cortex. The sensor and driver are brought onto the field and connected to the stabilizer bars and their capacitance is tested. The sensor is placed in the mastoid cavity so that its tip is just lateral to the body of the incus. The driver is placed parallel to the stapes crura with the tip, and thus lateral to the precoat on the stapes head (see **Fig. 1**). Gelfoam is placed around the sensor and driver bodies to prevent cement from entering the middle ear. The table is rotated away. Hydroxyapatite cement is placed in the mastoid cavity around the sensor and driver bodies (Video 6). The cement is allowed to cure/harden for 20 minutes.

Once the cement has hardened, ionomeric cement is placed around the driver tip, securing it to the stapes precoat. A small amount of ionomeric cement is placed around the sensor tip. After a few minutes, a neojoint is created by carefully freeing the sensor/cement from the incus body. The mastoid and middle ear are then flushed with saline, which is then vacuumed. A small piece of reflector tape is placed on the posterior crus of the stapes. The sensor and driver are then tested using the laser vibrometer; if either one is not working correctly, it might need to be revised. Once functioning correctly, the wires are cleaned and the sound processor/battery is connected (**Fig. 7**) and a system test is performed. The system tests assess displacement of the incus and stapes, which on average is approximately 100 nm,[7] and potential sources of feedback limiting device performance. The wound is then closed in layers using 2-0 Vicryl for the soft tissues over the sound processor and mastoid,

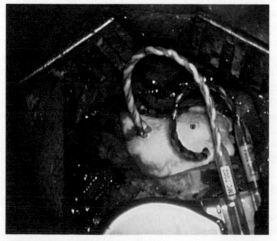

Fig. 7. Right Envoy Esteem completed surgery.

and 3-0 Vicryl in a subcuticular fashion for the skin. A long-acting local anesthetic is infiltrated into the incision line. A mastoid dressing is placed and the procedure is completed.

Potential Complications and Management

Because the procedure is one of the most complex in otology, only surgeons who have completed several training sessions are currently allowed to perform Esteem surgery. Many of the complications below will require termination of the surgical procedure, and therefore it is best to work in a slow and methodical fashion while performing the surgery to avoid complications. Injury to hair follicles when raising the skin flaps can result in areas of alopecia. Also, not drilling a deep enough well for the sound processor can cause a poor cosmetic result, because the processor may be very visible in patients with short hair. Mastoidectomy complications can include injury to the bony ear canal, sigmoid sinus, and tegmen. During the facial recess portion of the procedure, the incus buttress can be fractured, the ear canal can be entered, the tympanic membrane can be perforated, and the mastoid segment of the facial nerve and the horizontal semicircular canal can be injured.

Using the laser adds additional potential complications to this procedure. When using the laser to section the incus long process, a heat injury can occur to the tympanic segment of the facial nerve that may not be detected by the facial nerve monitor, and to the tympanic membrane, resulting in a burn or perforation. This complication is best avoided through keeping the middle ear packed with Gelfoam continuously moistened with saline.

The procedure also requires fine manipulation around the incus body (while creating the neojoint) and the stapes head (during cleaning and then placing the precoat). Injury to the incus can result in hypermobility or dislocation. When cleaning the stapes head, the annular ligament can become loosened and the stapes can even become dislocated, possibly resulting in sensorineural hearing loss, deafness, and dizziness.

Unique issues are also caused by the sensor, driver, and cement. The sensor and driver must be aligned perfectly for the device to work, and these may need to be repositioned or revised in the even the device does not work. The best way to prevent this complication is to check their position before cement application by repositioning the microscope several times and rechecking positions. It is also important to make sure the driver bellows movement is not limited by the facial ridge. When placing the cement to hold the sensor or driver in place, it can enter the middle ear or the housing of the sensor or driver. The sensor or driver may need to be removed and a new one placed, and any cement entering the middle ear would have to be removed. The cement should also be kept moist while drying because it can fracture. In this case, new cement would need to be placed in the crack.

When cementing the driver tip to the stapes precoat, it is important to completely cover the anterior portion of the driver. If the driver tip is not completely covered, the stapes displacement may be affected. If too much cement is applied to the stapes, a feedback bridge may occur between the stapes and incus remnant or the stapes and tympanic membrane. In these cases, the incus long process may need to be resected more and/or the stapes/driver connection may need to be redone.

If a functioning system cannot be implanted, the components may need to be removed. The stapes/driver connection can be disconnected using a right-angle pick or laser to heat and fracture the cement. The hydroxyapatite cement can then be curetted and/or drilled and the sensor and driver then removed. In this case, the ossicular chain can be reconstructed with the ionomeric cement.

POSTPROCEDURAL CARE
Medical Follow-up

Because the procedure is performed on an outpatient basis, patients go home after the procedure. Local patients are typically seen in the office 1 to 2 weeks after the procedure to check the incision and wound for signs of infection, hematoma or seroma, and wound dehiscence. Patients from out of state are contacted via phone the week after surgery, because the first follow-up appointment is generally scheduled at 6 to 8 weeks postoperatively in conjunction with activation of the device by audiology. Patients from out of state can also e-mail pictures of the wound if they have any concerns during the postoperative period.

Audiologic Follow-up

The first audiology appointment is generally performed at 6 to 8 weeks postoperatively. The gain is increased as much as possible, but usually maximal gain is not achievable at this point because resolving fluid in the mastoid and middle ear is typically present, causing feedback. One or two other appointments, generally at 2-month intervals, will allow the gain to be increased as the mastoid and middle ear fluid resolves.

REHABILITATION AND RECOVERY

Most patients will do very well once maximal gain is achieved at approximately 4 to 6 months after surgery, with high patient satisfaction. If issues occur with the performance of the device, the system allows testing of the sound processor to troubleshoot the device. Many of these issues can be resolved with reprogramming.

Similar to patients with cochlear implants, those who receive Envoy Esteem implants are not able to undergo MRI testing. Furthermore, the use of monopolar cautery near the device can cause it to malfunction. Patients are allowed to participate in water sports.

The sound processor/battery will generally last 4.5 to 9.0 years, depending on use. It can be replaced via a minor outpatient surgical procedure using local or general anesthesia, depending on patient preference. A portion of the incision in front of the sound processor is opened. The wires are carefully dissected and the leads are removed, cleaned, and placed in the new processor. The incision is then closed in layers.

SURGICAL AND HEARING OUTCOMES

Because the Envoy Esteem is a new device targeting a small patient population, few articles have been published on the subject. These articles are described in the next session. Because the device was approved by the US Food and Drug Administration in 2010, these studies are limited by small patient populations and limited follow-up. These studies generally compare patients with Esteem implants with those with best-fit hearing aids and not with those with other types of implantable hearing devices.

Bilateral Implantation

Patients who are very satisfied with the performance of their Esteem implant may elect to have their contralateral ear implanted. The surgeon should ascertain the patients has no active wound issues (eg, exposed wires, wound drainage) with the current Esteem before offering contralateral surgery. The surgeon should also assess the hearing in the contralateral ear to ensure it is stable and falls within the medical criteria, and confirm that the size of the mastoid cavity is adequate to accommodate the implant.

Costs Associated with the Envoy Esteem

For most patients undergoing Esteem implantation, commercial insurance carriers, Medicare, and Medicaid will not cover the device and/or surgical procedure. Costs associated with the procedure include the device and engineer support, anesthesia, surgical center time and materials, audiology, and surgical fees. Total costs for Esteem implantation in the United States average between $35,000 and $45,000 per ear. Implant centers offering the Esteem device may choose to work with organizations such as Care Credit (www.carecredit.com) to offer patients financing options.

CLINICAL RESULTS IN THE LITERATURE

The largest study to date by Kraus and colleagues[5] in 2011 assessed 57 patients with bilateral mild to severe sensorineural hearing loss with word recognition scores greater than 40% who underwent Envoy Esteem implantation. Hearing results with the Esteem were compared with preimplant baseline unaided and best-fit aided conditions. Speech reception thresholds improved from 41.2 to 29.4 dB, and the word recognition score at 50 dB improved from 46.3% to 68.9%. The study had 6 complications, including 2 wound infections (1 requiring device explanation), 1 delayed facial paralysis, and 3 revisions because of limited benefit. A smaller study by Shohet and colleagues[8] examined a series of 5 patients with profound sensorineural hearing loss who underwent Esteem implantation with 12 months of follow-up. Preoperative speech reception thresholds improved from an unaided 65 dB and aided 45 dB to 26 dB with the Esteem, and word recognition scores at 50 dB improved from an unaided 10% and aided 23% to 78% postoperatively.

REVISION SURGERY

The best way to decrease the need for revision surgery in these patients is to properly select the correct patients to implant. Patients with mild to moderate sensorineural hearing loss with good word recognition who have not given conventional high-power hearing aids an adequate trial are best served by doing so. At the other end of the spectrum, patients with severe or profound sensorineural hearing losses with word recognition scores less than 40% are best treated with cochlear implantation.

Patients who have undergone Esteem implantation and experienced limited benefit despite troubleshooting and reprogramming may be candidates for revision surgery, which can generally be undertaken using 2 approaches. Patients whose testing indicates a possible feedback bridge between the driver and tympanic membrane or between the driver and the incus remnant may be approached through a transcanal revision. Adhesions can be sharply resected and the tympanic membrane replaced. A drawback of this approach is that issues with the sensor or with the driver within the mastoid cavity cannot be addressed.

The other approach is a transmastoid revision through the initial incision. The sound processor is removed from its pocket and the sensor and driver leads are removed and their corresponding wires are carefully dissected. The leads are then connected for testing. The benefit of this approach is that the entire system can be inspected visually and tested, and issues can be addressed. Fibrous tissue around the sensor and/or driver can be removed until the device is working properly. The sensor neojoint can be redone if necessary. The sensor and/or the driver can be removed and replaced. Because the hydroxyapatite cement around the sensor and driver is likely osseointegrated at this point, the driver/stapes interface will need to be disrupted before any drilling of the cement can occur. In general, problems are more likely to occur with the driver than with the sensor. Patients who are initially doing very well at 6 months after implantation but then show decreased gain and/or increasing feedback may have scar tissue development impacting sensor and/or driver function. Patients with abundant fibrous tissue may even require device explanation. In these cases, the ossicular chain can be reconstructed with ionomeric cement. Once healed, these patients can have their hearing retested and may be able to again wear hearing aids or may be candidates for cochlear implantation. In a recently submitted study (Sappington JA and Marzo SJ, unpublished data, 2014) assessing 71 Esteem primary surgeries over a 3-year period, 9 patients required explanation for excessive scar tissue, biofilms, or infection. Twenty patients underwent either transmastoid or transcanal revision procedures with successful results. A total of 43 of these patients had complete preoperative and postoperative audiologic data. The preoperative unaided pure tone average was 63.4 dB and the postoperative pure tone average was 50.7 dB. The average gain was 9.9 dB, which was statistically significant.

SUMMARY

The Envoy Esteem is the first completely implantable hearing device. It is indicated for patients older than 18 years with stable moderate to severe sensorineural hearing losses with word discrimination scores greater than 40%. Patients undergoing implantation should have limited hearing benefit using best-fit hearing aids. The device is generally not covered by insurance companies. The surgical procedure is technically demanding and the best hearing results are typically seen at 6 months postoperatively. Complications with the device are uncommon. Finally, hearing results with the Esteem are generally better than those with hearing aids.

SUPPLEMENTARY DATA

Supplementary data related to this article can be found online at http://dx.doi.org/10.1016/j.otc.2014.08.006.

REFERENCES

1. National Institute on Deafness and other Communication Disorders. Quick Statistics. Available at: http://www.nidcd.nih.gov/health/statistics/Pages/quick.aspx. Accessed September 10, 2013.
2. Shargorodsky J, Curhan SG, Curhan GC, et al. Change in prevalence of hearing loss in US adolescents. JAMA 2010;204:722–8.
3. Chien W, Lin FR. Prevalence of hearing aid use among older adults in the United States. Arch Intern Med 2012;172(3):292–3.
4. Chen DA, Backous DD, Arriaga MA, et al. Phase 1 clinical trial results of the Envoy System: a totally implantable middle ear device for sensorineural hearing loss. Otolaryngol Head Neck Surg 2004;131:904–16.
5. Kraus EM, Shohet JA, Catalano PJ. Envoy Esteem Totally Implantable Hearing System: phase 2 trial, 1-year hearing results. Otolaryngol Head Neck Surg 2011; 145(1):100–9.
6. Envoy Medical Corporation. Premarket Approval Application. Available at: http://www.fda.gov/downloads/AdvisoryCommittees/CommitteesMeetingMaterials/MedicalDevices/MedicalDevicesAdvisoryCommittee/EarNoseandThroatDevicesPanel/UCM194412.pdf. Accessed October 1, 2013.

7. Seidman M, Standring RT, Ahsan S, et al. Normative data of incus and stapes displacement during middle ear surgery using laser Doppler vibrometry. Otol Neurotol 2013;34(9):1719–24.
8. Shohet JA, Kraus EM, Catalano PJ. Profound high-frequency sensorineural hearing loss treatment with a totally implantable hearing system. Otol Neurotol 2011; 32(9):1428–31.

Implantable Hearing Devices
The Ototronix MAXUM System

Stanley Pelosi, MD[a],*, Matthew L. Carlson, MD[b],
Michael E. Glasscock III, MD[b]

KEYWORDS

- Ototronix MAXUM • SOUNDTEC • Implantable hearing device
- Electromagnetic ear implant • Conventional hearing aid • Functional gain
- Word discrimination • Residual hearing

KEY POINTS

- The MAXUM system (Ototronix LLC, Houston, TX) is a semi-implantable hearing device that provides hearing-impaired patients with an alternative to conventional hearing aids.
- Patients implanted with the MAXUM system technology have demonstrated a functional gain in hearing significantly greater than that of conventional hearing aids.
- Patient questionnaire has shown a subjective reduction in acoustic feedback and the occlusion effect for MAXUM technology users relative to conventional hearing aids.
- The MAXUM system may be surgically implanted in a short procedure performed under local anesthesia, with a low risk of procedure-related adverse events.

INTRODUCTION

Hearing loss affects approximately 30 million people in the United States, including up to one-third of individuals older than 65 years.[1] An estimated 75% to 80% of people who could potentially benefit from hearing aids (HAs) do not seek amplification; of the patients who are fitted with HAs, many are poorly compliant in using them. Reasons for this lack of compliance include acoustic feedback/distortion, occlusion effect, ear canal discomfort/irritation, and social stigma.[2] Although new technologies have reduced some of these drawbacks, they have been largely unable to overcome the

Disclosures: Dr M.E. Glasscock is chairman of the Ototronix (Houston, TX) medical advisory board and has a minor equity position in Ototronix.
[a] Department of Otolaryngology, The New York Eye and Ear Infirmary, 310 East 14th Street, New York, NY 10003, USA; [b] Department of Otolaryngology, Vanderbilt University Medical Center, 7209 Medical Center East-South Tower, 1215 21st Avenue South, Nashville, TN 37232, USA
* Corresponding author.
E-mail address: spelosi@nyee.edu

Otolaryngol Clin N Am 47 (2014) 953–965
http://dx.doi.org/10.1016/j.otc.2014.08.003
0030-6665/14/$ – see front matter © 2014 Elsevier Inc. All rights reserved.

oto.theclinics.com

difficulties that many patients with conventional aids still face when listening in crowded, noisy environments.

Implantable and semi-implantable hearing devices (IHDs) have been developed as an option for patients who derive limited benefit from traditional HAs but who are not yet candidates for cochlear implants. All IHDs have in common the ability to provide amplification via a direct driver to the ossicles, which is stimulated to vibrate by either electromagnetic or piezoelectric energy. Because IHDs do not use a speaker to amplify ambient noise, they eliminate the acoustic feedback seen with conventional aids. The review of recent literature has suggested that IHDs can amplify sound as good or perhaps greater than conventional HAs.[3,4]

The Ototronix MAXUM system (Ototronix LLC, Houston, TX) is a semi-implantable device that amplifies sound using electromagnetic energy transferred from an external ear canal mold to an internal surgically implanted magnet. The system is based on technology that was previously marketed as the SOUNDTEC Direct Drive Hearing System (SOUNDTEC Inc, Oklahoma City, OK), which received approval from the Food and Drug Administration in 2001. Although the SOUNDTEC device used a behind-the-ear processor, the MAXUM system differs in that it has a combined digital sound processor and electromagnetic coil worn in the ear canal (known as the *integrated processor and coil* [IPC]). The internal component is the same for both devices and consists of a permanent magnetic implant attached to the ossicular chain.

Sound presented to the external component of the MAXUM system is received by the microphone, amplified, and processed into an electrical signal, which is then delivered to the electromagnetic coil in the ear canal mold. The charged coil then produces an electromagnetic field in the middle ear space, which stimulates the magnet attached to the incudostapedial (IS) joint. Vibrations of the magnet are synchronous to the original sound input, which are then transmitted to the stapes and on to the cochlea.

CANDIDACY FOR SURGERY

Candidates for the MAXUM system include adults 18 years of age and older with moderate to moderately severe sensorineural hearing loss (SNHL), ideally with a high-frequency pure tone average (1, 2, and 4 kHz) between 35 and 70 dB. A necessary prerequisite for candidacy is a normal conductive hearing system. Bone conduction thresholds should be within 10 dB of air conduction values, and word recognition scores should be 60% or better. Patients must have normal middle ear anatomy, no history of middle ear surgery, and no evidence of acute/chronic otitis media, retrocochlear lesions, or central auditory disorders.

PREOPERATIVE PLANNING, PREPARATION, AND COUNSELING

All patients should undergo a thorough otologic examination and audiometric evaluation before being considered for surgery. MRI can be helpful to exclude retrocochlear pathology in cases of asymmetric hearing loss, whereas computerized tomography can evaluate the extent of middle ear/mastoid pathology when the otologic examination suggests abnormalities. All candidates should be provided with other options for hearing rehabilitation, including the use of conventional HAs. Validated subjective questionnaires, such as the Hough Ear Institute Profile,[5,6] may reveal problems with conventional aids, including acoustic feedback, which can be reduced with an IHD. Additional counseling before surgery should ensure that patients have realistic expectations of the device advantages and limitations as well as a thorough understanding of surgical risks inherent to middle ear surgery.

The choice of ear to implant is based on several considerations. In patients with objective asymmetry in air conduction thresholds, word discrimination scores, or speech reception thresholds, the poorer-hearing ear is implanted first. When no objective difference is observed, the ear not used to talk on the telephone is chosen. If no preference exists, then patient choice alone is used as a deciding factor.

The size and shape of the external ear canal must be assessed before surgery to ensure functionality of the device. Before surgical implantation, a deep ear impression is taken. In order for the ear canal is able to accommodate the IPC, the following ear canal dimensions have been specified as a prerequisite for implantation: 20-mm canal length from aperture to medial canal, 4-mm width at the canal aperture, and 3-mm canal diameter from the second bend of the canal to the medial portion.[7]

OPERATIVE PROCEDURE

For most individuals, the MAXUM system is implanted under local anesthesia using a transcanal stapedectomy-type approach. Intravenous access is obtained, and oral and/or intravenous sedation is administered. Patients are positioned supine with the head resting on a foam cushion and tilted away from the surgeon. The surgical site is then prepped and draped so that monitoring of the facial nerve can take place. A mixture of 1% lidocaine with 1:30,000 epinephrine is used for pain control and hemostasis. Injections are made superiorly and inferiorly in the soft tissues of the cartilaginous ear canal and then more medially in the posterior vascular strip.

An incision is made along the posterior canal wall, and a tympanomeatal flap is elevated. The annulus of the tympanic membrane is identified and elevated out of its sulcus to enter the middle ear space. Posterosuperior bone of the medial bony canal is curetted, taking care not to injure the chorda tympani nerve. Bone should be removed until the IS joint, posterior stapes crura, and pyramidal process can be clearly visualized. The oval window niche and mobility of the ossicular chain are now evaluated, along with the position of the facial nerve. Attention is then directed toward the IS joint, the site of attachment of the MAXUM implant.

The implant magnet is composed of neodymium iron boron, housed in a titanium cylinder, and attached to an open wire-form ring (**Fig. 1**). The cylinder measures

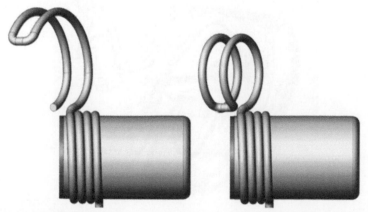

Fig. 1. The MAXUM split coil is shown in open and closed configuration. A 30° angle exists between the cylinder and the attachment coil to facilitate optimal implant alignment when attached to the IS joint. (*Courtesy of* Ototronix, Spring, TX; with permission.)

2 mm in length and 1.35 mm in diameter; the implant weighs 27 mg.[8] To minimize contamination of the implant, the surgeon should not directly handle the implant. Nonmagnetic MAXUM surgical instruments are available for implant handling during package removal and insertion, including a cylinder-holding forceps (**Fig. 2**) and/or a suction insertion tool, controlled by a foot pedal allowing the surgeon to vary suction strength (**Fig. 3**). Once the implant has been introduced to the middle ear, the open portion of the attachment coil is placed around the IS joint (**Fig. 4**). This coil is composed of nitinol, a memory alloy that, when exposed to heat, will form a closed coil around the IS joint. The attachment coil should not be manually crimped. One commercially available low-temperature heating device that may be used for closure of the coil is the SMart Piston Heating Device (Gyrus ENT, Stamford, CT, **Fig. 5**). A standard laser is also an option for coil closure. Although no specific manufacturer recommendations for laser settings exist, the similarity of the implant's nitinol material to the stapes SMart prosthesis suggests that the same laser settings may be used. One previously reported laser setting with the argon laser in SMart piston stapedotomy is 0.7 W with a pulse duration of 0.1 second.[9] Older versions of the implant used a full coil (**Fig. 6**), which required separation of the IS joint to secure the implant. Surgical technique with the full coil has previously been summarized.[10]

Several factors related to positioning of the implant will affect performance of the MAXUM system. The electromagnetic coil in the ear canal mold and the magnet should be aligned in a parallel manner in order to maximize the magnet's vibratory capabilities and resulting functional gain of the device.[8] To allow for optimal alignment, the implant is designed with a 30° angle between the cylinder and the attachment coil (see **Fig. 1**). If the implant is situated correctly, it will be parallel to the ear canal and the surgeon will see only the end of the cylinder but not the sides (**Fig. 7**).

Also important is the distance between the external coil and the internal magnet, with shorter distances creating a larger magnetic field. The attachment ring is designed to be off-center near the base of the magnet cylinder, thus positioning the magnet closer to the tympanic membrane. This design also reduces the likelihood

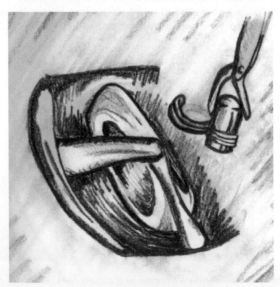

Fig. 2. The nonmagnetic MAXUM cylinder-holding forceps may be used to grasp the implant cylinder.

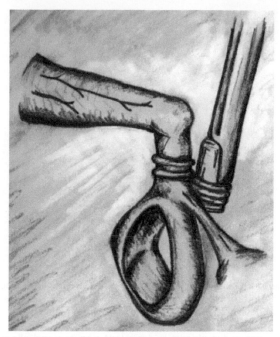

Fig. 3. The nonmagnetic MAXUM suction insertion tool may be used to grasp the cylinder. The surgeon can vary suction strength using a foot pedal attached to the insertion tool.

of implant contact with the promontory, which is important for unimpeded magnet vibration. In cases when a high promontory is present, it may also be necessary to rotate the cylinder to avoid contact. The cylinder can be rotated in any one of 3 positions (**Fig. 8**) to prevent promontory contact.

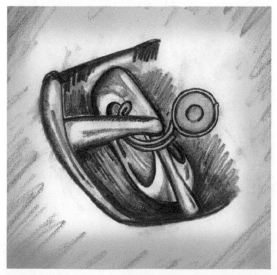

Fig. 4. The open portion of the attachment coil is placed around the IS joint.

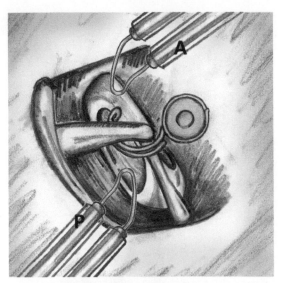

Fig. 5. A low-temperature heating device can be placed anterior (A) or posterior (P) to the attachment coil and used for closure of the coil. Shown in the image is a rendering of the SMart piston heating device. (Gyrus ENT, Stamford, CT.)

Once the attachment coil is closed and implant position and alignment have been confirmed, the implant is stabilized with an absorbable gelatin sponge (Gelfoam). Nonmagnetic instruments are then used to return the tympanomeatal flap to its normal position. If it is found that the implant touches or closely approximates the tympanic

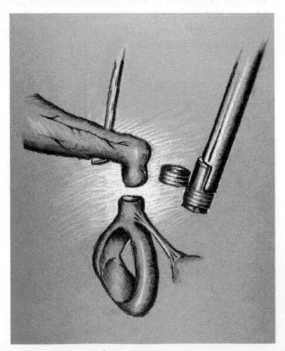

Fig. 6. The full coil version of the wire-form attachment ring requires separation of the IS joint.

Non-Optimal Alignment

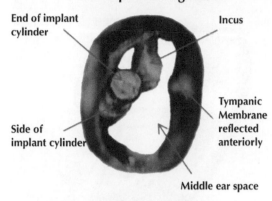

End of implant cylinder

Incus

Side of implant cylinder

Tympanic Membrane reflected anteriorly

Middle ear space

Optimal Alignment

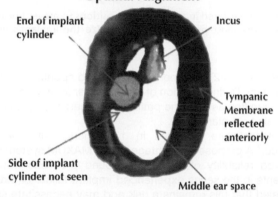

End of implant cylinder

Incus

Tympanic Membrane reflected anteriorly

Side of implant cylinder not seen

Middle ear space

Fig. 7. Correct positioning of the implant cylinder parallel to the ear canal will allow the surgeon to see only the end of the cylinder but not the sides.

membrane, placing a tragal cartilage graft just medial to the tympanic membrane may help prevent device extrusion. This cartilage graft can be harvested with a perichondrial sleeve, which in turn can be draped over the magnet to facilitate implant stabilization.[10] Although magnet contact with the rigid promontory should be avoided to prevent impairment of vibration, magnet contact with the cartilage/perichondrial graft and/or tympanic membrane should not significantly impede magnet vibration.

POTENTIAL COMPLICATIONS AND MANAGEMENT

All patient candidates should be counseled on the inherent risks of middle ear surgery, including the loss of residual hearing, infection, dizziness, taste changes, and facial nerve injury. Other perioperative risks may exist that are specific to the MAXUM system. The largest study reporting on adverse events associated with the technology used in the MAXUM system was a series of 103 patients implanted with the aforementioned SOUNDTEC Direct System device.[6] Perioperative events were relatively limited and most commonly included ear pain (n = 16), taste changes (n = 2), and tympanic

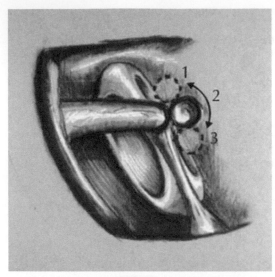

Fig. 8. The cylinder can be rotated in any one of 3 positions to prevent promontory contact. Usually, position 3 is the most preferable to maximize the implant's distance from the promontory.

membrane perforation (n = 2). One perforation closed spontaneously, and the other required myringoplasty. During creation of the deep ear impression, 7 patients developed small canal hematomas and one patient sustained a tympanic membrane perforation, which healed spontaneously.

External processor failure occurred in 13 patients with the behind-the-ear SOUNDTEC device.[7] A proposed advantage of the MAXUM system over older technology is improved reliability of the digital sound processor found in the IPC. Although no patients in the series experienced implant failure or extrusion, patients should be counseled that this remains a risk and may necessitate surgical revision.

MEDICAL AND AUDIOMETRIC FOLLOW-UP

Patients are discharged on the day of surgery; postoperative antibiotics are not routinely prescribed. Patients are instructed to follow similar precautions as other individuals undergoing middle ear surgery to reduce the likelihood of postoperative implant displacement. A list of postoperative instructions for MAXUM users is provided by the manufacturer and includes avoidance of nose blowing, exercise, straining, heavy lifting, and contact sports in the weeks after surgery.[7] Water precautions during the healing period are also recommended to reduce the risk of postoperative infection.

Patients are typically fitted with the IPC approximately 3 weeks after surgery, and device activation occurs at this time. Because the device provides a deep fit of the ear canal, occasionally patients may need to wait a few additional weeks before IPC fitting so as to ensure complete postsurgical healing. When not wearing the IPC, no water precautions exist once healing is complete, although the external device itself is not waterproof.

The IPC fitting process and software programming adjustments necessary to ensure functionality of the MAXUM system typically require 1 to 3 postoperative visits. During fitting, small adjustments in the shape of the IPC can be undertaken to optimize its alignment with the implanted magnet. The tip of the device is heat moldable and may be contoured based on the patients' individual anatomy, and the material has memory so that this process can be reversed and repeated if necessary.

Once an optimal fit of the IPC is obtained, additional digital programming adjustments can be performed at subsequent visits so as to provide maximal amplification and comfort for each individual patient. Postoperative audiometric evaluation is typically performed about 2 months after surgery.

PRECAUTIONS WITH THE MAXUM SYSTEM

The issue of MRI compatibility has been examined in the SOUNDTEC Direct System, which shares the same technology as the MAXUM. Both linear and torsional forces affect the implant in a magnetic field, with the latter being more significant and potentially leading to displacement of the implant and/or ossicular chain.[11] Also contributing to the MRI risk are heating of the magnet (creating the potential for surrounding tissue damage), implant demagnetization, and image distortion/degradation. Because of these risks, the official manufacturer recommendation is that patients with the MAXUM system should not undergo MRI or be in close proximity to magnetic fields.[7] To address the issue of patients in whom MRI is necessary, Hough and colleagues[6] initially suggested that the device may be removed under local anesthetic and reinserted after MRI has been completed. However, Dyer and colleagues[12] more recently reported that patients with the SOUNDTEC device may safely undergo low-strength MRI. This study showed no patient- or device-related complications in 11 patients with the SOUNDTEC device who underwent a total of 12 head, 1 shoulder, and 3 lumbar MRIs at a strength of 0.3 T.[12] To minimize MRI-related risks, Dyer and colleagues[12] recommended a protocol whereby the patient was positioned so that the implant and MRI static fields were oriented parallel and the head was placed in a lateral position (to minimize implant torque). Furthermore, the use of a fast spin echo sequence may reduce implant artifact and image degradation in the region of the implant.

Other manufacturer precautions have been described for patients with the MAXUM system. The split coil version of the MAXUM implant contains nickel, posing risk to patients with hypersensitivity reactions to this metal. The effects of radiation therapies, such as cobalt treatment or linear acceleration, on the MAXUM system are unknown. Electric currents applied to the body in procedures such as electroconvulsive therapy and diathermy may damage the implant or cause additional patient hearing loss; both are contraindicated in patients with the MAXUM system. Similarly, the manufacturer has recommended that monopolar cautery be avoided because of the risk of demagnetization and/or device malfunction. Although no studies have specifically examined the safety of monopolar cautery in IHDs, this has been investigated for cochlear implants, which have similar theoretic susceptibilities to electrical current. One cadaver study showed no changes in cochlear implant impedance, integrity testing, or intracochlear temperature following the application of monopolar cautery of up to 50 W in either the oral cavity or abdomen.[13] Although it may be tempting to extrapolate such results to IHDs, further study is needed with the MAXUM system before any definitive recommendations regarding safety with monopolar cautery can be made.

Use of the MAXUM system near any device that creates electromagnetic fields, including antitheft detectors and airport security devices, may cause sound distortion but should not be harmful to the implant or patients. Silverstein and colleagues[14] reported that patients experienced increased device vibration and noise in areas with surrounding magnetic fields (eg, near power lines, security systems). Similarly, radiofrequency identification systems (eg, keyless entry systems, toll roads) may occasionally interfere with the MAXUM system and cause abnormal sound perception. Finally, certain conventional HAs have been associated with sound distortion when using a cell phone, but the MAXUM system is generally considered to be compatible with cell phone technology.

OUTCOMES

Several studies have reported outcomes with the technology used in the MAXUM system; these are summarized in **Table 1**. The phase II trial by Hough and colleagues[6] demonstrated the SOUNDTEC device to provide an average functional gain of 7.9 dB at 500 to 4000 Hz relative to the patients' own optimally fit conventional HA. The HAs used by patients in this study exhibited considerable variability, including analog and digital processors as well as styles ranging from in-the-canal to behind-the-ear devices; consequently, it is unknown as to whether these conventional aids were indeed providing patients with maximal benefit. Roland and colleagues[5] reported a mean 9.9 dB functional gain over the patients' own optimally fit conventional HAs in a subset of 23 patients enrolled in the phase II trial, whereas Silverstein and colleagues[14] corroborated similar results when comparing the amplification provided by the SOUNDTEC device with the previously published values of conventional HA gain.

Word discrimination scores were assessed in each of the aforementioned series. Hough and colleagues[6] demonstrated a statistically significant 5.3% average improvement in speech discrimination scores with the SOUNDTEC device. Speech in noise scores was also higher relative to conventional aids, although this improvement did not reach statistical significance. In comparison, Roland and colleagues[5] found no significant differences in speech perception in quiet or noise, whereas Silverstein and colleagues[14] reported a mean 6% decline in word discrimination with the SOUNDTEC device compared with preoperative aided values.

Regarding residual hearing following implantation, Roland and colleagues[5] reported no significant change before and after implantation. The phase II trial demonstrated that average air conduction thresholds declined by 4 dB overall and by more than 10 dB in 10.5% of study participants.[6] Two factors may account for conductive hearing loss associated with the MAXUM system. Weighting of the ossicular chain by the implant, with resulting impairment of ossicular vibration, is one consideration. Also, because these patients were implanted with the older full coil, an additional conductive hearing loss is expected because of the temporary separation of the IS joint. Increased use of the split coil in future procedures may reduce the degree of conductive loss seen in some patients after surgery.

Variable degrees of SNHL have been reported following implantation. Hough and colleagues[6] reported an average decline in bone conduction thresholds of 1.1 dB, whereas Silverstein and colleagues[14] found that 21 patients experienced an average bone conduction threshold shift of 10 dB or greater.[14] SNHL may result from ossicular manipulation during magnet implantation that results in excessive perilymph vibrations and damage to the inner ear. Such a loss may in part account for the aforementioned decline in postoperative word discrimination scores reported by Silverstein and colleagues.[14]

Several studies have also reported subjective patient outcomes for the MAXUM system technology. Patient questionnaire results from Hough and colleagues[6] and Roland and colleagues[5] showed a statistically significant improvement in patient satisfaction as well as a significant reduction in acoustic feedback and occlusion effect compared with conventional HAs. In assessing the subjective benefit, Silverstein and

Table 1								
Clinical outcomes with technology used in the MAXUM system								
Study	n	Length of Follow-up (mo)	Control	Residual Hearing	Functional Gain	Speech Perception in Quiet	Speech Perception in Noise
Roland et al,[5] 2001	23	5	Conventional HA	NS	Mean 9.9 dB >HA at 250–4000 Hz[a]	NS	NS
Hough et al,[6] 2002	103	12	Conventional HA	• Mean 4 dB AC loss (NS) • Mean 1.1 dB BC loss (NS)	Mean 7.9 cB >HA at 500–4000 Hz[a]	Mean 5.3% improvement[a]	NS
Silverstein et al,[14] 2005	64	3	Conventional hearing aid	21 Patients with >10 dB mean BC loss	Mean 26 dB >postop unaided thresholds	Mean 6% decline (did not assess significance)	DNT

Abbreviations: AC, air conduction; BC, bone conduction; DNT, did not test; NS, no significant difference; postop, postoperative.
[a] Statistically significant difference.
Data from Refs.[5,6,14]

colleagues[14] reported that 55% of patients complained of magnet movement, necessitating device removal in certain instances (see the section on revision surgery below).

REVISION SURGERY

Silverstein and colleagues[14] discussed details of revision surgery for patients with the SOUNDTEC device. Three patients complaining of magnet motion underwent revision surgery for magnet stabilization with adipose tissue. Revision surgery entailed a transcanal approach under sedation and local anesthetic. Adipose tissue was obtained from the earlobe and placed adjacent to and around the magnet. Postoperatively, these patients were reported to experience symptom improvement. Four patients underwent device explantation because of dissatisfaction with the device and subsequently were able to successfully use conventional HAs. No studies have reported on ossicular erosion at the time of revision surgery. Other than adhesions and scarring inherent to any revision transcanal procedure, no special challenges are known to be associated with revision MAXUM surgery.

SUMMARY

The MAXUM system is a viable option for hearing amplification in patients seeking an alternative to conventional aids. Outcomes with the technology used in this device have demonstrated improved functional gain as well as reduced feedback and occlusion effect in comparison with HAs. More comprehensive data regarding long-term outcomes will help further define the value of the MAXUM system as an option for aural rehabilitation in the future.

REFERENCES

1. Kochkin S. Hearing loss population tops 31 million people. Hear Rev 2005;12:16–29.
2. Haynes DS, Young JA, Wanna GB, et al. Middle ear implantable hearing devices: an overview. Trends Amplif 2009;13:206–14.
3. Butler CL, Thavaneswaran P, Lee IH. Efficacy of the active middle-ear implant in patients with sensorineural hearing loss. J Laryngol Otol 2013;127(Suppl 2): S8–16.
4. Tysome JR, Moorthy R, Lee A, et al. Systematic review of middle ear implants: do they improve hearing as much as conventional hearing AIDS? Otol Neurotol 2010; 31:1369–75.
5. Roland PS, Shoup AG, Shea MC, et al. Verification of improved patient outcomes with a partially implantable hearing aid, the SOUNDTEC direct hearing system. Laryngoscope 2001;111:1682–6.
6. Hough JV, Matthews P, Wood MW, et al. Middle ear electromagnetic semi-implantable hearing device: results of the phase II SOUNDTEC direct system clinical trial. Otol Neurotol 2002;23:895–903.
7. Hough JV, Dyer RK, Glasscock ME. Surgeon's manual, Maxum system. Houston: Ototronix, LLC; 2012.
8. Hough JV, Dyer RK Jr, Matthews P, et al. Early clinical results: SOUNDTEC implantable hearing device phase II study. Laryngoscope 2001;111:1–8.
9. Harris JP, Gong S. Comparison of hearing results of nitinol SMART stapes piston prosthesis with conventional piston prostheses: postoperative results of nitinol stapes prosthesis. Otol Neurotol 2007;28:692–5.
10. Dyer K. The SOUNDTEC direct system: surgical technique. Cochlear Implants Int 2005;6(Suppl 1):69–72.

11. Dyer RK Jr, Dormer KJ, Hough JV, et al. Biomechanical influences of magnetic resonance imaging on the SOUNDTEC Direct System implant. Otolaryngol Head Neck Surg 2002;127:520–30.
12. Dyer RK Jr, Nakmali D, Dormer KJ. Magnetic resonance imaging compatibility and safety of the SOUNDTEC direct system. Laryngoscope 2006;116:1321–33.
13. Jeyakumar A, Wilson M, Sorrel JE, et al. Monopolar cautery and adverse effects on cochlear implants. JAMA Otolaryngol Head Neck Surg 2013;139:694–7.
14. Silverstein H, Atkins J, Thompson JH Jr, et al. Experience with the SOUNDTEC implantable hearing aid. Otol Neurotol 2005;26:211–7.

Otologics Active Middle Ear Implants

Herman A. Jenkins, MD*, Kristin Uhler, PhD

KEYWORDS

- Middle ear transducer • Carina • Active middle ear prosthesis • Cochlear
- Otologics

KEY POINTS

- Active middle ear implants increase our rehabilitation armamentarium available in situations in which traditional amplification is not adequate.
- The adoption of traditional amplification remains a problem for a variety of reasons.
- Use of an implantable middle ear prosthesis requires a major commitment from the patients, families, surgeon, audiologist, and educator, particularly if and when future candidacy expands to include the young pediatric age range.
- The reliability of implantable devices has greatly improved with newer generations of the implants, but failures do still occur.
- The best results are achieved in settings with trained surgeons, audiologists, and educators working together with implant patients.

 A video of Otologics surgery accompanies this article at http://www.oto.theclinics.com/

INTRODUCTION

The World Health Organization estimates that approximately 600 million people are affected with hearing loss worldwide. Of these, 250 million suffer from moderate to severe hearing losses. In the United States, 28 million Americans have hearing loss severe enough to impact communications. The magnitude of the problem worldwide is overwhelming in how one begins to rehabilitate these hard-of-hearing and deaf individuals.

Traditional hearing aids have seen major advances in recent years, both in fidelity of sound and cosmetic appearance. Although most of the hard-of-hearing population could benefit from traditional amplification, only 15% to 20 % actually use these

Department of Otolaryngology, University of Colorado, School of Medicine, 12631 East 17th Avenue, B205, Aurora, CO 80045, USA
* Corresponding author.
E-mail address: herman.jenkins@ucdenver.edu

Otolaryngol Clin N Am 47 (2014) 967–978
http://dx.doi.org/10.1016/j.otc.2014.08.007
0030-6665/14/$ – see front matter © 2014 Elsevier Inc. All rights reserved.

devices. Even in the severely affected group with marked compromise of communication skills, only 55% use hearing aids.[1,2] All health care workers are familiar with the many rationales for not wearing amplification devices.[3] Aesthetic appearance, cost, discomfort in wearing, restriction in activities, quality of sound, and medical conditions (such as canal deformity, chronic external otitis, and chronic middle ear disease) are common complaints from our patients. This lack of adoption of even new hearing aid technology has encouraged manufacturers to develop a new line of technology that is implantable to alleviate these common problems.

The active middle ear prostheses use semi-implantable and fully implantable technology to stimulate the inner ear. In the past decade, rapid advances have been made in the field; these are available in the market place for patients with mild to severe hearing losses. Implantable devices fall into 4 general categories: acoustic osseointegrated prostheses, active middle ear prostheses, cochlear implants, and auditory brainstem implants, along with hybrid devices. This article centers on the semi-implantable and fully implantable Otologics LLC devices, now Cochlear Corporation (Sydney, Australia) active middle ear prostheses.

REQUIREMENT FOR ACTIVE MIDDLE EAR PROSTHESES

Semi-implantable and fully implantable active middle ear prostheses all require common components: a sensory pick up mechanism, processing electronics, a power source, communication system, and a stimulator. The approach has varied with companies, but the needs remain the same. Although technology in implantable devices has made major strides, challenges remain in developing microphone technology, a translating stimulator, and an implantable power source.

In semi-implantable devices, the microphone, processing electronics, and power source can all be maintained externally with information and power being delivered transcutaneously via a telecommunication coil or magnetic induction. In these devices, many of the technological problems have been solved; the results rely more on signal processing than microphone and battery technology.

In fully implantable devices, these challenges have slowed down the introduction of this technology into the hard-of-hearing patient population. The development of a fully implantable microphone has been one of the major stumbling blocks in all implantable hearing devices. A microphone must be sensitive to ambient sounds, ignoring biologic noises while implanted under a layer of skin and subcutaneous tissue. Adding 6 mm of soft tissue over a microphone decreases its effectiveness by tenfold, thus requiring an enlargement of the microphone system by tenfold. The sensitivity to biological noises and skull vibrations, as during voicing or chewing, is increased 100 fold under 6 mm of soft tissue. Thus, some cushioning of the microphone is required to temper the biological sounds.

Battery technology has made major advances in the past decade. The power source needs to be capable of delivering at least 16 hours of device use without recharging to be an effective amplifier for patients. It should be safe and provide sufficient power for all operating conditions over the life of the implant. It is now feasible to have a small battery sufficient to drive active middle ear prostheses for 24 plus hours between charges. Larger batteries similar to cardiac pacemaker technology can last 5 to 7 years without recharging before requiring replacement.

Electrodes in cochlear implants have now been implanted in patients with devices lasting for several decades. This development is a relatively straightforward technological development when compared with an active middle ear prosthesis. Stimulating the intact inner ear requires a translating system that converts sound energy into movements of the ossicular chain or tympanic membrane. These constantly moving devices must be engineered to survive in a hostile biological system with host protective mechanisms, such as inflammation and fibrosis chronically attempting to wall off the foreign body and protect the host.

Manufacturers have used a variety of techniques to solve these problems. Success has been achieved, though often at the sacrifice of other elements of the system. One must appreciate that we are still in the initial developmental stages, similar to the period of very early cochlear implants; great developments are here and yet to come.

The Otologics LLC has transferred their intellectual properties for the hearing devices to Cochlear Corporation. All the work reported next used devices supplied by Otologics LLC; therefore, the name *Otologics* is used in referring to the device. This device should not be confused with the present Cochlear Corporation products, such as the Baha or Cochlear Nucleus cochlear implants (Cochlear Corporation, Sydney, Australia). Cochlear Corporation is currently marketing the latest generation of the Carina (Cochlear Boulder, Otologics LLC, Boulder CO) in Europe and South America.

OTOLOGICS MIDDLE EAR TRANSDUCER (SEMI-IMPLANTABLE)

The Otologics Middle Ear Transducer (MET), has a button external processor that provides power and sound stimulation through a transcutaneous coil to the implanted digital electronics hermetically sealed package and transducer (**Fig. 1**). The stimulator is an electromagnetic transducer that is mounted in a titanium bracket anchored to the mastoid bone with the transducer tip loaded against the body of the incus (**Fig. 2**). Power to the internal device and sound signals are transmitted transcutaneously through a radio coil from the external button to the implant digital electronics processing the sound and controlling movement of the transducer. Sound induces translation

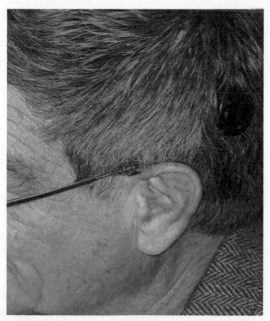

Fig. 1. External button processor of the Otologics semi-implantable MET. (*Courtesy of* Cochlear Boulder, Boulder, CO; with permission.)

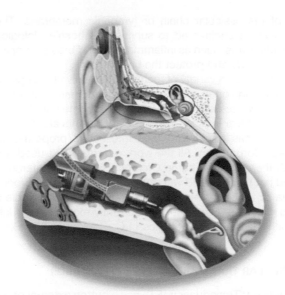

Fig. 2. The Otologics semi-implantable MET anchoring in the temporal bone. (*Courtesy of* Cochlear Boulder, Boulder, CO; with permission.)

of the transducer with resultant stimulation of the ossicular chain through incus movement.

OTOLOGICS CARINA (FULLY IMPLANTABLE)

The Otologics Carina has a traditional microphone implanted in the cortical bone of the mastoid and attached to the implant canister through a dependent lead. The hermetically sealed implant canister contains the electronics package and battery (**Fig. 3**). A traditional communication coil used in other implant technology along with a magnet allows recharging the battery and adjustments of software algorithms, along with volume of sound. The transducer is electromagnetically driven and is loaded against the body of the incus, mechanically translating to stimulate the ossicular chain.

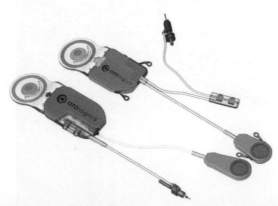

Fig. 3. Otologics fully implantable Carina implant. Left is previous generation reported on in this article. Right is the current generation being implanted in Europe. (*Courtesy of* Cochlear Boulder, Boulder, CO; with permission.)

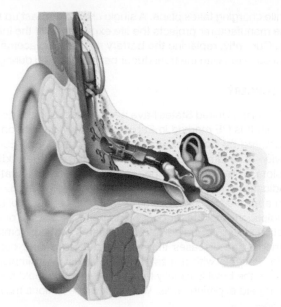

Fig. 4. An implanted Otologics Carina with anchoring in the mastoid. (*Courtesy of* Cochlear Boulder, Boulder, CO; with permission.)

It is anchored securely to the mastoid via a titanium bracket, and the degree of incus loading is adjusted by a feedback loop system to assure sustained contact with maximal compliance of the system (**Fig. 4**). As the pickup sensor is located remotely to the external and middle ear, the ossicular chain is not disrupted.

Patients recharge the device daily. A mobile charging unit consists of a mobile charger that is continuously charged in a base connected to an electrical current. The mobile charger is then removed, and the communication antenna is magnetically attached to the implanted communication coil to recharge the implant (**Fig. 5**). Charging requires approximately 1 hour or less per day to maintain the longevity of the internal nickel-cadmium battery. Patients can remain mobile and continue to

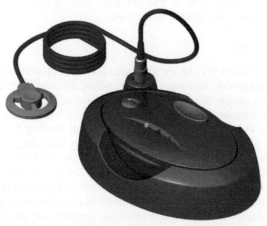

Fig. 5. Charging unit, base, and telecommunication coil. (*Courtesy of* Cochlear Boulder, Boulder, CO; with permission.)

use the device while charging takes place. A single charge can last up to 30 plus hours of device use. The manufacturer projects the life expectancy of the internal battery to be 12 to 15 years. Currently, replacing the battery requires replacement of the microphone and implant canister, with the transducer being detached during the procedure.

CANDIDACY FOR SURGERY

Current clinical trials in the United States have been closed, and the device is not available for implantation. It is CE marked in Europe, and new-generation Carina devices are being manufactured by Cochlear Boulder for implantation in Europe and South America. The device is recommended for adults who meet the audiometric criteria (see later discussion). The device may be used in a variety of situations in patients with no contraindications for surgery or middle ear implantation. Candidacy has been expanded in approved locations for sensorineural, conductive, and mixed hearing loss. Contraindications include retrocochlear, central auditory, or functional hearing loss. Implantation is also contraindicated in patients with concomitant disease, as persistent otitis media and diseases that require a 2- to 3-hour general anesthetic would not be safe. Patients with a mastoid cavity have been implanted in Europe, and an obliteration of the bowl is usually required. Patients should have had previous conventional hearing aid experience, as, without it, expectations may be too high for the implanted device.

PREOPERATIVE PLANNING AND PREPARATION

Patients undergo preoperative assessment of hearing, including pure tones, middle ear impedance, and speech testing. It is important that they have had a reasonable, generally 3 months, trial of use of an appropriately fitted hearing aid. In patients failing hearing aid trials or needing to use a hearing aid in hostile situations, such as swimming or exercise, the fully implantable device would be an option. Patients are counseled as to the surgery and the possibility that performance most likely will be at approximately the same level as their conventional hearing aid. There is a slim possibility of decreased hearing from injury to the ossicular chain. Bleeding and infections are infrequent. A computed tomography scan of the temporal bones is obtained preoperatively to ensure there is normal anatomy that would allow implantation of the transducer in the attic area of the mastoid. With use in many situations, the candidacy criteria have been greatly expanded.

AUDIOMETRIC CRITERIA

For the semi-implantable MET device, the inclusion criteria were adults (>18 years of age), bilateral sensorineural hearing loss of postlingual onset, greater than 40% on monosyllabic words, stable hearing loss, and realistic expectations of device benefit.

For the fully implantable device, the inclusion criteria were similar: bilaterally symmetric hearing loss in the mild to severe sensorineural hearing loss range, monosyllabic word scores greater than 40% at 80 dB hearing level (HL) or 40 dB sensation level (SL), postlingual onset of hearing loss that is stable, and worn hearing aids verified to match targets for prescriptive fitting method (Desired Sensation Level [DSL] or National Acoustic Laboratories [NAL]) for a minimum of 3 months before entering the study. **Fig. 6** illustrates the hearing range of potential candidates for implantation. Preoperative and postoperative evaluation included unaided air and bone conduction, monaural aided and unaided thresholds in the sound field, Consonant Nucleus Consonant (CNC) and Bamford-Kowal-Bench Sentence in Noise (BKB-SIN) word

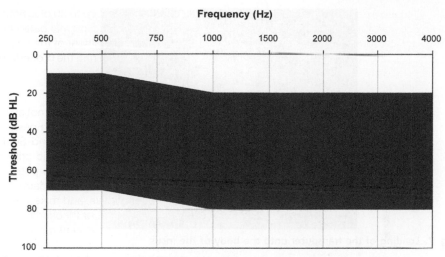

Fig. 6. The candidacy range for Otologics Carina and MET implantation.

discrimination, Abbreviated Profile of Hearing Aid Benefit (APHAB), and Otologics subjective questionnaire.

SURGICAL TECHNIQUE

Patients are positioned in a supine head lateral position, and the periauricular area is prepped and draped in a sterile fashion. An incision is made in the postauricular sulcus, and the upper limb is extended posteriorly for approximately 2 cm. The mastoid and squamosa of the temporal bone are exposed. An atticotomy is performed to permit visualization of the head of the malleus and body of the incus. The bone overlying the epitympanum and the canal wall are thinned to give adequate view and approach for mounting the transducer. A titanium bracket is firmly mounted in the attic, positioned such that the transducer will be directed toward the body of the incus. A countersink is performed in the posterior aspects of the mastoid for the microphone and in the posterior parietal area for implantation of the hermetically sealed canister. The transducer is positioned in the bracket and advanced manually to within 1 to 2 mm of the body of the incus, being in a perpendicular position as much as possible. An O-ring is used to tighten the transducer firmly in position, and a microadjust wrench advances the tip of the transducer against the body of the incus. A feedback transducer-loading assistant is used to measure when adequate loading has been achieved without overloading (**Fig. 7**). The transducer lead is attached to the implant canister and tested to ensure microphone response. The skin is closed in a standard fashion.

Procedural Approach

Video 1 demonstrates the Otologics procedure.

POTENTIAL COMPLICATIONS AND MANAGEMENT

As this is a minimally invasive mastoid procedure, the procedure has limited complications. Chief among these is disarticulation of the incus or drilling on the incus with attendant conductive or sensorineural loss. If hearing loss occurs from injury to the ossicular chain, the chain is explored and repaired as needed. A hemotympanum is routinely seen after surgery and does not require intervention. This procedure is

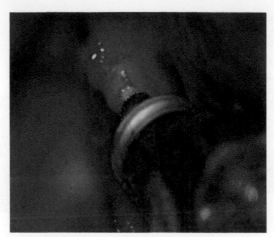

Fig. 7. Loading of the transducer onto the body of the incus.

unlikely to cause vertigo, change in taste, or facial weakness, as the surgery does not intrude deeply into the mastoid.

POSTPROCEDURAL CARE

Patients are asked to remove their dressing after 24 hours and may begin showering with washing their hair after 48 hours. They return for follow-up at 1 week or earlier if the patients are experiencing symptoms, such as marked swelling or drainage from the wound. The wound is checked for healing problems or signs of infection. Two months are allowed to pass before programming of the device. Early programming requires frequent adjustments as the skin overlying the implanted microphone is thinning, becoming more adherent to the device with improved transmission of sound through the microphone.

AUDIOLOGY FOLLOW-UP

Subjects were evaluated preoperatively with the test battery (see audiometric criteria). The device was activated 8 weeks postoperatively; evaluations were repeated at 3, 6, and 12 months after the implantation. Programming of the device was done following the assessment protocol using the Otologics Otofit software. Each time the device was programmed, an in situ audiogram was measured. After the audiogram was measured, microphone measurements were conducted to determine feedback of the microphone. Desired sensation level was the prescriptive gain method used.[4] Programming was similar to a traditional hearing aid with the exception that the authors were not able to obtain real ear measurements with this system. In addition to programming, data logging of the device use and device diagnostics were obtained at each visit. These diagnostic measures included battery/current drain and impedance of the transducer.

REHABILITATION AND RECOVERY

Once implanted, patients must refrain from undergoing an MRI as an internal magnet drives the transducer, and this would be damaged or displaced. The manufacturer has not verified any conditions in which an MRI would be safe; if the patients' health mandates an MRI, the entire system must be removed. The fully implanted system can be safely used in hostile environments for conventional hearing aids, such as water sports, vigorous exercise, and dirty work environments. Scuba diving may result in changes to the processing program when under water pressure, but this would theoretically return to normal after completion of the dive. However, the depth of safe dives or use of hyperbaric oxygen therapy has not been clearly established in implanted patients; these activities are currently contraindicated with both the partially and fully implanted systems. Use of monopolar cautery around the device and in the head and neck area is contraindicated, as is ionizing radiation of the overlying skin. Monopolar cautery can be used for surgeons operating below the clavicles.

SURGICAL AND HEARING OUTCOMES

The authors have taken part in clinical trials in the United States for the semi-implantable and fully implantable systems. The results reported here represent their experience with only references to studies outside the United States.

Audiological Outcome Measures

For the semi-implantable MET device, there was minimal change in unaided air conduction thresholds consistent with ossicular chain loading and no change in bone conduction.[5] However, the thresholds improved at most frequencies by 12 months; the authors attribute the change in thresholds to the healing process. The functional gain of prostheses when compared with conventional hearing aids indicated more functional gain with the active prostheses compared with the conventional aids, predominately in the high versus low frequencies.

Direct comparisons were made between the preoperative walk-in hearing aids and the postoperative Otologics MET. When preoperative CNC word scores were compared with the 12-month postoperative CNC word scores, there was not a significant difference. Hearing aids were programmed to meet prescriptive gain targets. The patients with the most severe losses perceived greater perceived benefit with the MET ossicular stimulator, documented by CNC scores and APHAB.

Clinical trials in the United States of the Otologics Carina showed no changes in the aided and unaided pure tone measures with implantation. Word discrimination on CNC and BKB-SIN was equivalent. Further analysis revealed that there was a relationship between preoperative and postoperative CNC word scores. Additionally, there was a negative relationship between pure tone average and CNC word scores. Specifically, as pure tone average increased (ie, poorer hearing), CNC word scores were poorer. Results were noted to improve with the maturation of the wound providing better contact with the microphone through thinning of the overlying skin. APHAB and subjective questionnaires showed APHAB scores revealed a significant improvement in benefit on the ease of communication, background noise, and reverberation at 3 months; background noise and reverberant environments at 6 months; and background noise at 12 months. The Otologics-developed questionnaires completed preoperatively and postoperatively showed a definite preference for the device in improvement of hearing, quality of sound, clearness of tones, and naturalness of sound, with preferences lasting over the year of the study (Uhler K, Jenkins HA. Otologics fully implantable active middle ear prostheses; phase IIb clinical trial results. Submitted for publication).[6,7]

FUTURE INDICATIONS FOR CONDUCTIVE AND MIXED HEARING LOSS

Although implantation of active middle ear prostheses represents a challenge in sensorineural loss, conductive and mixed loss offers even greater challenges. Lupo and colleagues[8] addressed some of these issues in an animal model using the *Chinchilla lanigera*. Using the Otologics MET transducer, they demonstrated that direct mechanical stimulation of the round window by an active middle ear transducer produced inner ear and cortical responses that were comparable with acoustic input. **Fig. 8** illustrates the compound action potential (CAP) in the chinchilla for the 3 experimental conditions. Fixation of the stapes resulted in a mild threshold shift of the cochlear microphonics and compound action potential in these animals similar to other studies in the human with stapes fixation and congenital absence of the oval window. However, the magnitude of the threshold shift expected was lower in the stapes fixation condition; the investigators speculated that other phenomenon may exist to explain this finding, such as a third window effect.

Human cadaveric temporal bone studies showed that improved laser Doppler vibrometer-measured stapes velocities could be obtained by drilling the lip of bone sheltering the round window membrane, using smaller probe tips, interposed tissue between the prostheses and the round window membrane and improved coupling of the prostheses to the incus using more stable clips closer to the stapes. No change was noted in the angle of stimulation of the stapes.[9-15]

The fully implantable Carina is now used clinically for conductive and mixed hearing loss with a variety of implantation sites, including the round window and footplate. The device is CE marked for this purpose in Europe and South America. Long-term results have demonstrated the utility of this device and its long-term stability. The transducer tip may be changed to fit the situation (ie, a ball for round window and a clip or bellow for stapes stimulation). Significant improvement in speech and pure tones has been reported from multiples sites throughout Europe.[16,17]

REVISION SURGERY

As of writing this article, 12 patients have been explanted from the phase IIb study, and 4 patients have been explanted from the phase I study. Explantation in phase I was performed for battery failure, which was detected early after implantation use was begun. In phase IIb, 2 were explanted for poor performance, 8 for device failures, 1 for infection, and 1 for recurrent shocking sensations. These patients were covered under a Food and Drug Administration protocol; they were not eligible for revision or reimplantation surgery, only explantation. The present generation that is being implanted outside the United States has now been used for more than 3 years, and device failure has not been an issue.

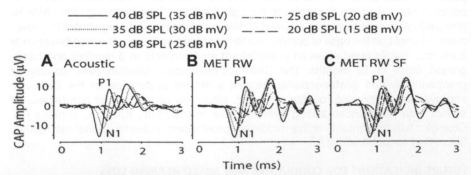

Fig. 8. Compound action potential (CAP) measured in the *Chinchilla langeria* in response to acoustic, round window (RW) MET, and round window MET with stapes fixation (SF). Curves in each plot represent different intensities of stimulation.

Revision surgery may be needed in implant failure or in decreased battery life. The old incision may be reopened and the components identified. The transducer lead may be separated from the implant canister and either the transducer or the implant canister and microphone removed as needed. If the transducer needs to be replaced, the transducer tip must be withdrawn from the body of the incus to prevent ossicular damage before removal from the mounting bracket. If implanted for some time, scar tissue occurs around the mounting bracket and often must be removed with the transducer. Scar tissue is rarely seen around the incus body and distal tip of the transducer.

Removal of the canister and microphone may be done after separating the transducer lead. This removal is easily accomplished with the new generation in use. The leads must be dissected carefully from the dense surrounding scar tissue, which is often difficult to do without damage to the microphone and transducer leads. If this were to occur, an entirely new device would have to be implanted.

SUMMARY

Active middle ear implants increase our rehabilitation armamentarium available in situations in which traditional amplification is not adequate. The adoption of traditional amplification remains a problem for a variety of reasons. The use of an implantable middle ear prosthesis requires a major commitment from the patients, families, surgeon, audiologist, and educator, particularly if and when future candidacy expands to include the young pediatric age range. The reliability of implantable devices has greatly improved with newer generations of the implants, but failures do still occur. The best results are achieved in settings with trained surgeons, audiologists, and educators working together with implant patients. All must gain expertise in the nuances of these devices.

The last 3 decades have been exciting in the explosion of new implant technology to improve communication skills. One must remain careful in candidate selection and long-term monitoring of outcomes.

SUPPLEMENTARY DATA

Supplementary data related to this article can be found online at http://dx.doi.org/10.1016/j.otc.2014.08.007.

REFERENCES

1. Snik FM, Cremers WR. First audiometric results with the Vibrant Soundbridge, a semi-implantable hearing device for sensorineural hearing loss. Audiology 1999; 38:335–8.
2. Popelka MM, Cruickshanks KJ, Wiley TL, et al. Low prevalence of hearing aid use among older adults with hearing loss: the epidemiology of hearing loss study. J Am Geriatr Soc 1998;46(9):1075–8.
3. Kochkin S. MarkeTrack VIII: the key influencing factors in hearing aid purchase intent: what factors would most likely lead non-adapters to purchase hearing aids? Hearing Review 2012;19(3):12–25.
4. Bagatto M, Moodie S, Scollie S, et al. Clinical protocols for hearing instrument fitting in desired sensation level methods. Trends Amplif 2005;9(4):199–226.
5. Jenkins HA, Niparko KK, Slattery WH, et al. Otologics Middle Ear Transducer™ (MET™) ossicular stimulator: performance results with varying degrees of sensorineural hearing loss. Acta Otolaryngol 2004;124:391–4.

6. Jenkins HA, Uhler K, Lupo VK, et al. Otologics middle ear system phase IIb clinical trial: preliminary results. In: Proceedings of the 7th Asia Pacific Symposium on Cochlear Implants and Related Sciences. Singapore: Medimond SRL; 2009. p. 51–56.

7. Zwartenkot JW, Hashemi J, Cremers CW, et al. Active middle ear implantation for patients with sensorineural hearing loss and external otitis: long-term outcome in patient satisfaction. Otol Neurotol 2013;34(5):855–61.

8. Lupo JE, Koka K, Holland NJ, et al. Prospective electrophysiological findings of round window stimulation in a model of experimentally-induced stapes fixation. Otol Neurotol 2009;30:1215–24.

9. Deveze A, Koka K, Jenkins HA, et al. Techniques to improve the efficiency of a middle ear implant: effect of different methods of coupling to the ossicular chain. Otol Neurotol 2013;34:158–66.

10. Kolka K, Holland NJ, Lupo JE, et al. Electrocochleographic and mechanical assessment of round window stimulation with an active middle ear prosthesis. Hear Res 2010;260:128–37.

11. Tringali S, Koka K, Deveze A, et al. Round window membrane implantation with an active middle ear implant: a study of the effects on performance of round window exposure and transducer tip diameter in human cadaveric temporal bones. Audiol Neurotol 2010;15:291–302.

12. Deveze A, Koka K, Tringali S, et al. Active middle ear implant application in case of stapes fixation: a temporal bone study. Otol Neurotol 2010;31:1027–34.

13. Tringali S, Koka K, Deveze A, et al. Intraoperative adjustments to optimize active middle ear implant performance. Acta Otolaryngol 2011;131:27–35.

14. Lupo JE, Koka K, Hyde BJ, et al. Physiologic assessment of active middle ear implant coupling to the round window in Chinchilla lanigera membrane. Otolaryngol Head Neck Surg 2011;145(4):641–7.

15. Lupo JE, Koka K, Jenkins HA, et al. Third-window vibroplasty with an active middle ear implant: assessment of physiologic responses in a model of stapes fixation in Chinchilla lanigera. Otol Neurotol 2012;33:425–31.

16. Martin C, Deveze A, Richard C, et al. European results with totally implantable Carina placed on the round window: 2-year follow-up. Otol Neurotol 2009;30(8):1196–203.

17. Lefebvre PP, Martin C, Dubreuil C, et al. A pilot study of the safety and performance of the Otologics fully implantable hearing device: transducing sounds via the round window membrane to the inner ear. Audiol Neurotol 2009;14(3):172–80.

Index

Note: Page numbers of article titles are in **boldface** type.

Otolaryngol Clin N Am 47 (2014) 979–982
http://dx.doi.org/10.1016/S0030-6665(14)00144-3
0030-6665/14/$ – see front matter © 2014 Elsevier Inc. All rights reserved.

United States Postal Service

Statement of Ownership, Management, and Circulation
(All Periodicals Publications Except Requestor Publications)

1. Publication Title	2. Publication Number								3. Filing Date
Otolaryngologic Clinics of North America	4	6	6	-	5	5	0		9/14/14

4. Issue Frequency	5. Number of Issues Published Annually	6. Annual Subscription Price
Feb, Apr, Jun, Aug, Oct, Dec	6	$365.00

7. Complete Mailing Address of Known Office of Publication (Not printer) (Street, city, county, state, and ZIP+4®)

Elsevier Inc.
360 Park Avenue South
New York, NY 10010-1710

Contact Person
Stephen R. Bushing
Telephone (Include area code)
215-239-3688

8. Complete Mailing Address of Headquarters or General Business Office of Publisher (Not printer)

Elsevier Inc., 360 Park Avenue South, New York, NY 10010-1710

9. Full Names and Complete Mailing Addresses of Publisher, Editor, and Managing Editor (Do not leave blank)

Publisher (Name and complete mailing address)

Linda Belfus, Elsevier Inc., 1600 John F. Kennedy Blvd., Suite 1800, Philadelphia, PA 19103-2899

Editor (Name and complete mailing address)

Joanne Husovski, Elsevier Inc., 1600 John F. Kennedy Blvd., Suite 1800, Philadelphia, PA 19103-2899

Managing Editor (Name and complete mailing address)

Adrianne Brigido, Elsevier Inc., 1600 John F. Kennedy Blvd., Suite 1800, Philadelphia, PA 19103-2899

10. Owner (Do not leave blank. If the publication is owned by a corporation, give the name and address of the corporation immediately followed by the names and addresses of all stockholders owning or holding 1 percent or more of the total amount of stock. If not owned by a corporation, give the names and addresses of the individual owners. If owned by a partnership or other unincorporated firm, give its name and address as well as those of each individual owner. If the publication is published by a nonprofit organization, give its name and address.)

Full Name	Complete Mailing Address
Wholly owned subsidiary of	1600 John F. Kennedy Blvd., Ste. 1800
Reed/Elsevier, US holdings	Philadelphia, PA 19103-2899

11. Known Bondholders, Mortgagees, and Other Security Holders Owning or Holding 1 Percent or More of Total Amount of Bonds, Mortgages, or Other Securities. If none, check box   ☐ None

Full Name	Complete Mailing Address
N/A	

12. Tax Status (For completion by nonprofit organizations authorized to mail at nonprofit rates) (Check one)
The purpose, function, and nonprofit status of this organization and the exempt status for federal income tax purposes:
☐ Has Not Changed During Preceding 12 Months
☐ Has Changed During Preceding 12 Months (Publisher must submit explanation of change with this statement)

PS Form 3526, August 2012 (Page 1 of 3 (Instructions Page 3)) PSN 7530-01-000-9931 PRIVACY NOTICE: See our Privacy policy in www.usps.com

---

13. Publication Title		14. Issue Date for Circulation Data Below
Otolaryngologic Clinics of North America		June 2014

15. Extent and Nature of Circulation		Average No. Copies Each Issue During Preceding 12 Months	No. Copies of Single Issue Published Nearest to Filing Date
a. Total Number of Copies (Net press run)		1,231	1,226
b. Paid Circulation (By Mail and Outside the Mail)	(1) Mailed Outside-County Paid Subscriptions Stated on PS Form 3541. (Include paid distribution above nominal rate, advertiser's proof copies, and exchange copies)	603	669
	(2) Mailed In-County Paid Subscriptions Stated on PS Form 3541 (Include paid distribution above nominal rate, advertiser's proof copies, and exchange copies)		
	(3) Paid Distribution Outside the Mails Including Sales Through Dealers and Carriers, Street Vendors, Counter Sales, and Other Paid Distribution Outside USPS®	334	285
	(4) Paid Distribution by Other Classes Mailed Through the USPS (e.g. First-Class Mail®)		
c. Total Paid Distribution (Sum of 15b (1), (2), (3), and (4))	▶	937	954
d. Free or Nominal Rate Distribution (By Mail and Outside the Mail)	(1) Free or Nominal Rate Outside-County Copies Included on PS Form 3541	36	37
	(2) Free or Nominal Rate In-County Copies Included on PS Form 3541		
	(3) Free or Nominal Rate Copies Mailed at Other Classes Through the USPS (e.g. First-Class Mail)		
	(4) Free or Nominal Rate Distribution Outside the Mail (Carriers or other means)		
e. Total Free or Nominal Rate Distribution (Sum of 15d (1), (2), (3) and (4))	▶	36	37
f. Total Distribution (Sum of 15c and 15e)	▶	973	991
g. Copies not Distributed (See instructions to publishers #4 (page #3))	▶	258	235
h. Total (Sum of 15f and g)	▶	1,231	1,226
i. Percent Paid (15c divided by 15f times 100)	▶	96.30%	96.27%

16. Total circulation includes electronic copies. Report circulation on PS Form 3526-X worksheet.

17. Publication of Statement of Ownership
If the publication is a general publication, publication of this statement is required. Will be printed in the December 2014 issue of this publication.

18. Signature and Title of Editor, Publisher, Business Manager, or Owner

Stephen R. Bushing – Inventory Distribution Coordinator

Date: September 14, 2014

I certify that all information furnished on this form is true and complete. I understand that anyone who furnishes false or misleading information on this form or who omits material or information requested on the form may be subject to criminal sanctions (including fines and imprisonment) and/or civil sanctions (including civil penalties).

PS Form 3526, August 2012 (Page 2 of 3)

Moving?

Make sure your subscription moves with you!

To notify us of your new address, find your **Clinics Account Number** (located on your mailing label above your name), and contact customer service at:

Email: journalscustomerservice-usa@elsevier.com

800-654-2452 (subscribers in the U.S. & Canada)
314-447-8871 (subscribers outside of the U.S. & Canada)

Fax number: 314-447-8029

Elsevier Health Sciences Division
Subscription Customer Service
3251 Riverport Lane
Maryland Heights, MO 63043

Printed and bound by CPI Group (UK) Ltd, Croydon, CR0 4YY

03/10/2024

01040486-0015